WATER AND WASTE

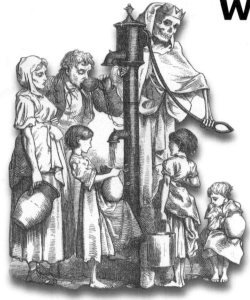

First published in 2009 by Middlesex University Press

Copyright © Jim Lewis

ISBN 978 1 904750 86 4

A CIP catalogue record for this book is available from The British Library

Design by Helen Taylor

Maps by Alice Gadney of Silver7 Mapping Ltd

Printed in the UK by Ashford Colour Press

Middlesex University Press
The Burroughs
Hendon
London NW4 4BT

Tel: +44 (0)20 8411 4162
Fax: +44 (0)20 8411 4167

www.mupress.co.uk

WATER AND WASTE

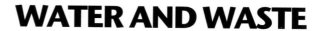

four hundred years of
health improvements
in the Lea Valley

Jim Lewis

Jim Lewis

&
Middlesex
University
PRESS

FOREWORD

LondonWaste Ltd is proud to support this second book in the Lea Valley series, *Water and Waste*. The company's flagship site is a 43-acre EcoPark in Edmonton North London, located on the A406 North Circular. Owned and run by LondonWaste, it is one of the capital's largest recycling, composting and recovery parks of its type, dealing with the daily creation of rubbish in some of the most environmentally friendly ways yet devised. This helps to lower the earth's carbon footprint by reclaiming useful materials that would have otherwise gone to landfill.

The perception of what "waste" is has changed and led the company to look closely at the three Rs: Reduce, Reuse and Recycle – with disposal as the last resort. LondonWaste Ltd continues to develop and extend its services to meet these challenges, and is committed to the principle of sustainable waste management. The company recycles, composts and recovers value, in the form of energy, from what's left over.

A great deal of thought has gone into the evolution of these services, which are unique in their entirety. The company is proud of what has been achieved, excited about plans for the future, and hopes that in the process you too will be inspired and realise the value of integrated waste management.

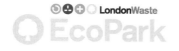

DEDICATION

This book is dedicated to my family and also to
my late mother and father, Leonora Maud Lewis
and Walter Harry Portman Lewis.

ABOUT THE AUTHOR

Dr Jim Lewis has spent most of his career in the consumer electronics industry, apart from a three-year spell in the Royal Air Force servicing airborne and ground wireless communications equipment. When working in the Lea Valley for Thorn EMI Ferguson he represented the company abroad on several occasions and was involved in the exchange of manufacturing technology. Currently he is a Consultant to Terry Farrell & Partners on the historical development of London's Lea Valley and a Workers' Educational Association (WEA) tutor teaching industrial history. He also teaches students within the Community Programme who have learning difficulties. A freelance writer, researcher and broadcaster for his specialist subject – London's Lea Valley – he also has a genuine passion for encouraging partnership projects within the local community, which in the long term are planned to help stimulate social and economic regeneration. Dr Lewis is married with four grown-up children and lives in Lincolnshire.

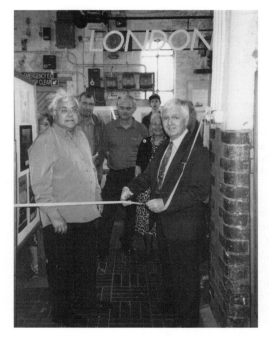

The author Dr Jim Lewis cutting the ribbon, with the Director of the Pump House Steam & Transport Museum Trust, Lindsay Collier MA, to open a special exhibition commemorating the 90th anniversary of the birth of the Associated Equipment Company (AEC), Walthamstow, the company responsible for the founding of London Transport (now Transport for London). Lindsay Collier and the Pump House Steam & Transport Museum Trust are responsible for designing and promoting the *Lea Valley Experience* project.

SERIES ACKNOWLEDGEMENTS

The author wishes to thank the following organisations, companies and societies for their encouragement, support and advice and for supplying many of the illustrations within this book:

Alexandra Palace and Park Trust, Wood Green, London
BAE Systems, Farnborough, Hampshire
Bishopsgate Institute, London
Black & Ethnic Minority Business Association, Walthamstow, London
BOC Process Plants, Edmonton, London
Brooklands Museum, Weybridge, Surrey
Bruce Castle Museum, Tottenham, London
Civix, Exton Street, London
Corporation of Trinity House, Tower Hill, London
Cuffley Industrial Heritage Society, Cuffley, Hertfordshire
Edmonton Hundred Historical Society, Enfield, Middlesex
Enfield Archaeological Society, Enfield, Middlesex
Enfield Business Centre, Enfield, Middlesex
Enfield Energy Centre Limited, Enfield, Middlesex
Enfield Enterprise Agency, Enfield, Middlesex
Enfield Local History Unit, Enfield, Middlesex
English Heritage, Blandford Street, London
Epping Forest Museum, Waltham Abbey, Essex
Greater London Record Office, Northampton Road, London
Gunpowder Mills Study Group, Guildford, Surrey
Guy & Wright Ltd., Green Tye, Hertfordshire
Hackney Society, Hackney, London
Harper Collins Publishers, Hammersmith, London
Hawker Siddeley Power Transformers, Walthamstow, London
Historical Publications Ltd., Barnsbury, London
Hornsey Historical Society, Hornsey, London
House of Lords Record Office, Westminster, London
Imperial War Museum, Duxford, Cambridgeshire
Institution of Civil Engineers, George Street, London
Institution of Engineering and Technology, Savoy Place, London
Institution of Mechanical Engineers, Birdcage Walk, London
Jewish Museum, Finchley, London
John Higgs, Freelance Historian, Fairford, Gloucestershire
Johnson Matthey, Enfield, Middlesex
Lea Valley Growers Association, Cheshunt, Hertfordshire
Lee Valley Business and Innovation Centre, Enfield, Middlesex
Lee Valley Regional Park Authority, Enfield, Middlesex
London Borough of Enfield, Enfield, Middlesex
London Borough of Haringey, Haringey, London
London Borough of Newham, East Ham, London
London Borough of Waltham Forest, Walthamstow, London
London Lee Valley Partnership Limited, Great Eastern Street, London
London Organising Committee of the Olympic & Paralympic Games, Canary Wharf, London
London Waste Ltd, Edmonton, London
Lotus Engineering, Hethel, Norwich, Norfolk
Marconi Archive, Oxford University Library Services, Oxford, Oxfordshire

Markfield Beam Engine & Museum, Tottenham, London
Midland Publishing Limited, Earl Shilton, Leicester
Ministry of Defence Library, Royal Armouries, Leeds, Yorkshire
Museum of London, London Wall, London
National Archive, Kew, Richmond, Surrey
National Army Museum, Chelsea, London
National Maritime Museum, Greenwich, London
National Portrait Gallery, London
Natural History Museum, Kensington, London
Navtech Systems Ltd., Market Harborough, Leicestershire
New River Action Group, Hornsey, London
Newham Local History Library, Stratford, London
North London Strategic Alliance, Wood Green, London
Perkins Group, Leyton, London
Phillips Auctioneers & Valuers, New Bond Street, London
Potters Bar Historical Society, Potters Bar, Hertfordshire
Pump House Steam & Transport Museum, Walthamstow, London
RCHME Cambridge, (National Monuments Record), Cambridge, Cambridgeshire
Reuters Limited, Fleet Street, London
River Lea Tidal Mill Trust, Bromley-by-Bow, London
Royal Air Force Museum, Hendon, London
Royal Commission on Historic Manuscripts, Quality Court, Chancery Lane, London
Royal Society of Chemistry, Burlington House, London
Royal Television Society, Holborn Hall, London
Science Museum, Kensington, London
Scout Association, Chingford, Essex
Southgate District Civic Trust, Southgate, London
Speedway Museum, Broxbourne, Hertfordshire
Stratford City Challenge, Stratford, London
Tesco, Cheshunt, Hertfordshire
Thames Water, Reading, Berkshire
Thorn EMI Archive, Hayes, Middlesex
Tower Hamlets Local History Library, Tower Hamlets, London
University of Leicester Space Research Group, Leicester, Leicestershire
Upper Lee Valley Partnership, Tottenham Hale, London
Valley Grown Nurseries, Nazeing, Essex
Vauxhall Heritage, Luton, Bedfordshire
Eric Verdon-Roe, grandson of Alliott Verdon-Roe
Vestry House Museum, Walthamstow, London
Waltham Abbey Royal Gunpowder Mills Company Ltd., Waltham Abbey, Essex
Walthamstow Amateur Cine Video Club, Walthamstow, London
WEA, London District, Luke Street, London
Wordsworth Editions, Ware, Hertfordshire

While many individuals have freely given their knowledge, some unknowingly, which has contributed greatly to the production of this series of books, I have, on a number of occasions paid special tribute to certain people in the footnotes of various chapters.

I could not let the occasion pass without recording my sincere thanks to my wife Jenny for her superb editorial skills and outstanding patience. The author freely admits that this voluntary sacrifice on Jenny's part has comprehensively tested the cement that holds our wonderful marriage together.

AUTHOR'S NOTE

Events such as the Olympics can be brought into our homes and workplaces from the host country as they take place through the power of electronic communication – radio, television, the Internet and satellite broadcasts. The technology that allowed this to happen was first discovered and developed at Ponders End, Enfield in London's Lea Valley.

In November 1904, after much experiment, Professor Ambrose Fleming registered his patent for the diode valve, the world's first thermionic device. This inspired invention not only paved the way for today's multimedia electronics industry, but also created the delivery platform for space travel, e-mail and the Internet, not to mention computers.

Thirty-two years after Fleming's invention, in November 1936, the world's first high-definition public service television broadcasts were transmitted by the BBC from Alexandra Palace, positioned on the crest of the Lea Valley's western slopes.

Centring the 2012 Olympic and Paralympic Games in London's Lea Valley will provide a unique opportunity to remind the world that it was the development of electronic communication within the region that has allowed the participating nations to share the message of peace and friendship.

Jim Lewis

CONTENTS

INTRODUCTION

It is probably fair to say that authors who research interesting and little-known historical subjects tend to resist the requests of their readers to produce yet another book highlighting new facts. Then, as in my case, the pressure becomes too great and the research bullet has to be bitten. Once the decision is made there is no turning back and the author is faced with months, sometimes years, of archive research to follow up reader leads and to see if sufficient material exists in a particular subject area to construct an interesting and worthwhile story. While the prospect of the challenge at first may appear daunting, once fully committed and immersed in the work the excitement level builds and it is particularly satisfying when new information comes to light.

In my last three books, I invited readers, particularly teachers and school children, to get involved in Lea Valley projects and also to take on the role of detectives to discover if more interesting stories existed about the region. Some schools and universities rose to the challenge and on a number of occasions I was invited to become involved and also to act as a Lea Valley tour guide. It is occasions like these that make writing doubly rewarding.

Due to considerable local interest, and also the requests by many retailers for reprints of earlier material, the author has been persuaded to deviate from the intentions of the original format used in my earlier Lea Valley books, that of keeping chapters deliberately short, and for this new series I shall include a fuller treatment of many of the subjects. Therefore, it is intended to give each book in the series a particular theme. In this way it is hoped that that the readers' requests will be largely satisfied and also a greater insight into the developments of the region will be achieved.

I have been greatly encouraged to be quoted by prominent writers and broadcasters such as Ian Sinclair and also to receive letters from Dr Adam Hart-Davis saying "I had no idea that the great George Parker Bidder was, no less, 'the maker of modern West Ham'. I told the story in the wilds of Moretonhampstead." The BBC newscaster Mike Embly, once referred to me as the "Lea Valley alarm clock" as

I appear to wake people up to the historic significance of the region. These compliments make the long hours in front of a computer screen and the many years of archive research seem worthwhile and this encourages me to discover and write more about the Lea Valley, its entrepreneurs and its world firsts. Perhaps, sometime in the future the region will no longer be Britain's best-kept secret.

As I am mindful that the forthcoming Olympics will bring many people to the Lea Valley from around the world, who will want to learn a little more about the region, I have decided to include some stories to attract those readers with broader interests beyond that of the subject of industrial heritage.

Jim Lewis

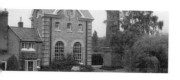

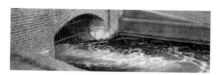

1. THE NEW RIVER, FROM ANCIENT TO MODERN – GOING WITH THE FLOW

An imaginative scheme to bring fresh drinking water to the City of London from springs situated north of the metropolis at Amwell and Chadwell in Hertfordshire, a distance of approximately twenty miles, began on 21 April 1609. After several acts of Parliament concerned with bringing water to London, a rather dilatory approach to such schemes by the Corporation, and progress slowed seemingly by high cost, a proposal put forward by Hugh Myddelton (later Sir) to fund and manage the venture was accepted formally, perhaps enthusiastically, on 28 March 1609.

Myddelton was born at Galch Hill near Denbigh, in or about the year 1555. He came from a large family of nine brothers and seven

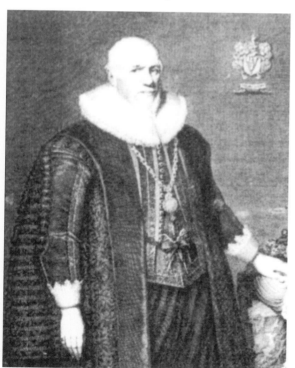

Sir Hugh Myddelton who, with King James I, put up the money to construct the New River.

sisters. His father Richard, who had been Governor of Denbigh Castle, died in 1575. His mother Jane had departed this life some ten years earlier in 1565. Hugh started his working career apprenticed to the Goldsmiths' Company and it would seem that part of his employment included banking and money changing. Between the years 1603 and 1628, he had been returned as Member of Parliament for the Borough of Denbigh on six occasions. It is probably fair to say that, had Hugh lived today, he would be labelled a venture capitalist and risk taker. Before Myddelton, Edmund Colthurst of Bath, Somersetshire had proposed a scheme to bring water from Hertfordshire to London but seems to have lacked the financial wherewithal to carry it through. When Myddelton undertook the task to finance and construct the new waterway, Colthurst was taken on as a partner and appointed

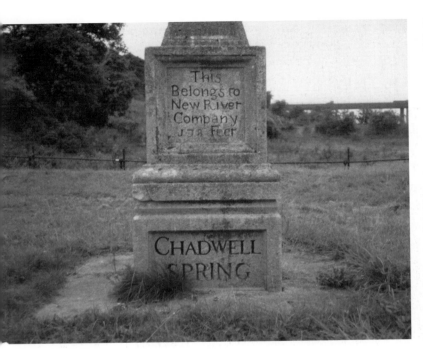

Chadwell Spring, the original source of the New River in 1609.

to manage the project, which should be seen as a sizeable civil engineering undertaking.

The plan for the construction of the New River, as it became known, was to follow closely the hundred-foot contour along the western slopes of the Lea Valley, the destination being a storage pond or reservoir which was to be dug at Islington. Deciding on this route for the river effectively doubled the distance the water had to travel from twenty to almost forty miles. However, what is so staggering about this project, which must be seen in the context of the day as a considerable feat of engineering, is that the channel dug from Hertfordshire brought water to the City by gravity only. In Britain, at that time, the use of pumps for shifting water was relatively rare. Only crude measuring instruments would have been available to the surveyors to complete their work like the "water level", used to plot the River's course along the hundred-foot contour. The labourers employed to dig the channel would have relied on picks and shovels to move the tons of earth and on occasions they would have been assisted by horses. In spite of all these technological difficulties, the workforce was able to achieve an astounding accuracy of construction as the average fall of water to Islington was only 5.5 inches (14cm) per mile.

Although construction of the New River was held up for almost two years due to disputes with landowners over the amount of

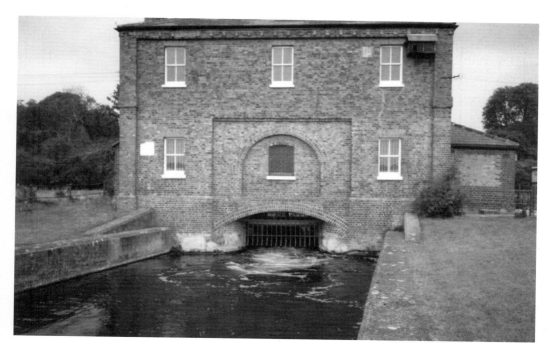

The New Gauge built in 1856 to replace the wooden gauge which regulated the flow of water from the River Lea. Water intake from the Lea to feed the New River is 22.2 million gallons daily.

compensation to be paid, the work was finally completed when the course was extended to Islington in April 1613. The official opening ceremony took place on 29 September that year with much celebration. Attending the celebrations were the then Lord Mayor, Sir John Swynnerton, Hugh Myddelton, and his brother the Lord Mayor elect, along with many other important people. Around sixty labourers dressed in their Sunday best shouldered their tools to parade around the round pond at Islington and, as might be expected on such occasions, many complimentary speeches were given. Eventually, the sluice gates were opened and trumpeters and drummers marked the occasion with a cacophony of sound as the water, which had journeyed from the chalk beds of the Chilterns via the springs of Amwell and Chadwell in Hertfordshire, flowed finally into the storage area of the round pond.

Considering the problems which had to be overcome, the speed of the waterway's completion is truly remarkable. It is recorded that 157 bridges spanned the river, which generally flowed north to south. However, there were many streams to negotiate which ran west to east across the valley carrying land drainage water. To reduce the risk of possible contamination to the clean water in the New River, these streams were allowed to follow their natural course towards the River Lea by being taken beneath the line of the new channel rather than being taken across the waterway in some form of aqueduct.

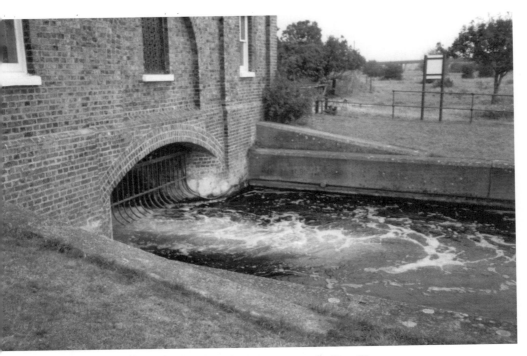

The New Gauge feeding water from the River Lea into the New River.

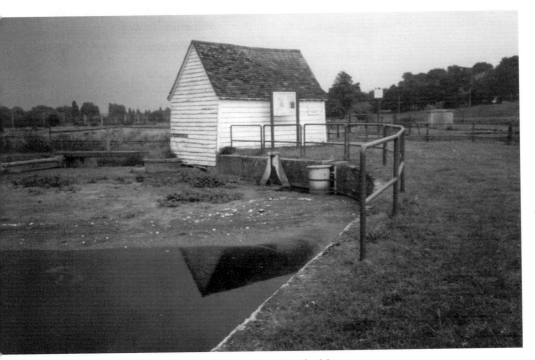

White House Sluice on the New River at Ware, Hertfordshire.

The Marble Gauge, erected in 1770, which formerly controlled the amount of water from the Manifold Ditch (the former course of the River Lea) to the New River.

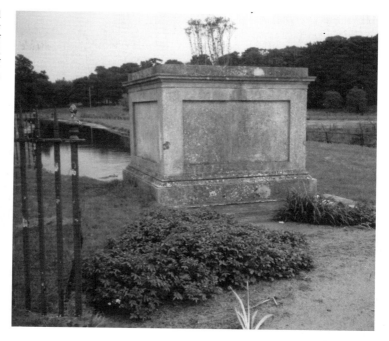

By today's standards, the sum of £18,525 to employ around six hundred workmen to construct the forty miles of New River that was ten foot wide with bridges, aqueducts and underground tunnels would appear to be an absolute bargain. But at the beginning of the seventeenth century this was a substantial sum for Myddelton to risk on a single venture. In fact, the holdups caused by the landowners trying to negotiate better prices put a considerable strain on Myddelton's finances and caused him to place his house on the market for sale. King James I finally came to the project's rescue but, for his contribution, he demanded a half share in future profits. Interestingly, in 1607, the King had exchanged his Hatfield estate in Hertfordshire with Robert Cecil's Theobalds Palace and estate near Cheshunt. Could it be that the line of the New River through the grounds of Theobalds Palace might have influenced the King in his decision to save the project? Arguably, the course of the waterway through his new acquisition was a factor as King James was soon to issue a decree urging the landowners not to hinder the River's future progress.

At the time when the New River was dug, Islington was effectively a village set in open country and situated approximately one hundred feet above the level of the River Thames. The spot chosen for the storage pond was quite deliberate, taking advantage of the natural fall of the land which gently sloped towards the City. This made water distribution relatively easy and it was possible, under gravity, to pipe water to the height of the second floor of some houses. In the early seventeenth century it would only have been the rich who could afford the luxury of piped water; poor people had to rely on their supplies from pumps, streams, the River Thames and the "water carriers" who plied their trade around the City. The "carriers" took their water from the same public sources as the majority of Londoner's and the impurity of this supply was often the cause of diseases like cholera and typhoid – although, at the time, the connections between drinking water and health were not generally understood by the population at large.

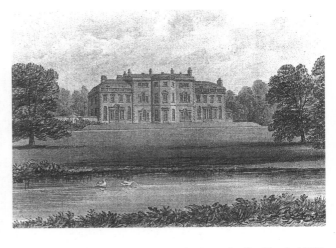

A picture by Buckler (c.1830) of Theobalds House. In the foreground is a section of the New River.

By today's standards, water distribution by the New River Company was rather crude. The main conduits were positioned above ground, sometimes on trestles, and were constructed from drilled sections of elm tree trunks. Each section was joined to the next by creating a friction joint secured with an iron ring. One end of a section was made to fit the next by shaping the mating piece like the sharpened end of a pencil. Individual house supplies were taken from the wooden main via a small-bore lead pipe which was usually terminated with a swan-necked cock for drawing off the water.

While those who benefited from this new method of water distribution were no doubt overjoyed, the system was very inefficient. Early in the nineteenth century, when several miles of wooden pipe were buried underground, it was reported that there

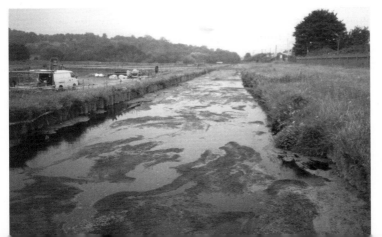

Looking north along the line of the New River from the Hornsey Pumping Station in north London.

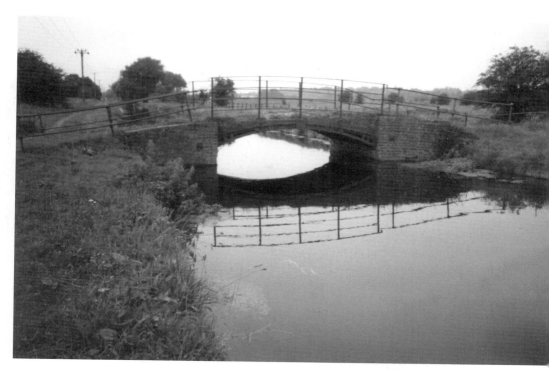

Bridge across the New River
at Ware in Hertfordshire.

were losses from the supply of twenty-five percent, attributed to leaks from pipes alone. However, it would be unwise to be too critical, considering the primitive nature of this early technology, as it has been reported only recently that losses of water from leaking pipes in some regions of Britain have been as high as forty percent. And of course, sections of elm log supported above ground on a trestle base would have been an open invitation to those of a mind to drill a small hole, under the cover of darkness, and so extract clean water to sell or use for personal consumption.

As the population of London increased, so did the demand for fresh drinking water. Over the years the New River saw many modifications to increase and quicken the flow into London. Bends were straightened, wells were dug, reservoirs were built and pumps installed. Today, when trying to trace the original route of the New River, it will be noticed that much has been filled in. However, due to sustained pressure from environmentally conscious community groups, a considerable amount of this ancient waterway has been saved and Thames Water has financed a public footpath with accompanying information boards along much of its length.

Today, some of the remaining sections of the New River form an integral and important part of a much larger and complex system of reservoirs, treatment works, pumping stations and filter beds

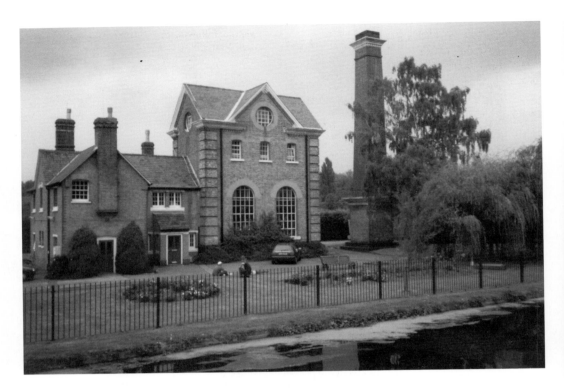

stretching along much of the length of the Lea Valley. In recent years, a scheme was completed to take water from the New River to re-charge the region's depleted aquifer, effectively connecting the ancient artefact to Thames Water's state-of-the-art London Ring Main (TWRM) which tunnels through the London clay at an average depth of forty metres below the metropolis. Incidentally, the depth of the Ring Main was chosen so as not to interfere with the London Transport Underground system and also other services like sewers, water mains and underground cables.

Building the eighty kilometre Ring Main first began in 1988 and was completed in 1993. Water within the Main's 2.54 metre diameter concrete pipe is not pumped but flows by gravity assisted by pressure from the ground level service reservoirs; this design has saved using considerable amounts of energy. Some twenty service shafts are connected to the Main where water can be fed to the various treatment works around London. Also, it is possible to recharge the Main through these service shafts from surface pumping stations positioned around the system. The initial cost of the project was in the order of £28 million but the work is still continuing with southern and northern extensions due for completion in 2009. This latter section will make the connection between the site of the former New River Head at Islington and

Broadmead Pumping Station constructed 1880, on the New River at Ware in Hertfordshire. The building is Grade II listed and modern electric pumps now lift the water from the aquifer to recharge the River.

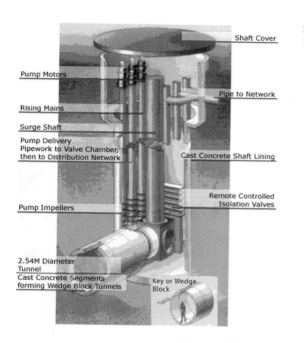

Shaft Cover

Pump Motors

Pipe to Network

Rising Mains

Surge Shaft

Pump Delivery
Pipework to Valve Chamber,
then to Distribution Network

Cast Concrete Shaft Lining

Remote Controlled
Isolation Valves

Pump Impellers

2.54M Diameter
Tunnel

Cast Concrete Segments
forming Wedge Block Tunnels

Key or Wedge
Block

Sectional drawing of a Thames Water
Ring Main pump-out shaft.

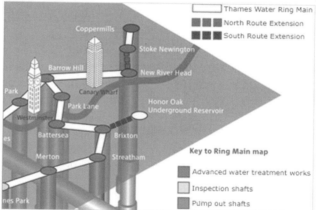

Diagram showing Thames
Water's northern Ring Main
extension.

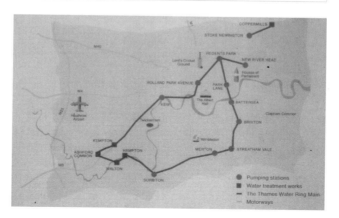

A plan showing the route of
the Thames Water Ring Main.

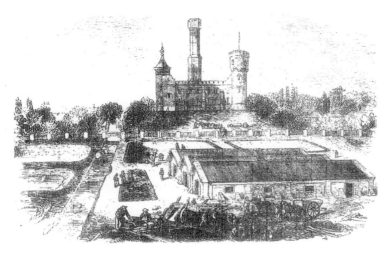

A mid-nineteenth-century engraving of Chadwell Mylne's pumping station and filter beds at Stoke Newington. The pump house is now home to the Castle Climbing Centre.

the New River pumping station and reservoirs at Stoke Newington, designed by the architect and civil engineer, William Chadwell Mylne (1781–1863).

Who could have imagined that four hundred years after the completion of the New River, the citizens of London would still be deriving benefit from the water brought to them by the remarkable skills and achievements of those early engineers and surveyors who designed and planned the waterway? Also, we should not forget the backbreaking contribution made by the labourers, who through sweat and hard manual toil shifted hundreds of tons of earth in digging the course of the river.

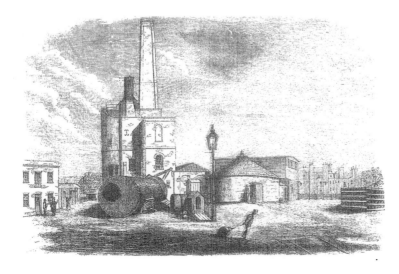

An engraving of Smeaton's extended engine house at New River Head, built c.1820 to accommodate a more powerful Boulton & Watt engine.

REFERENCES

Author unknown, "London's Water Supply in the 21st Century", a strategy for water treatment and trunk distribution, published by Thames Water, February 1986.

Cosh, Mary, *An Historical Walk Along the New River*, Islington Archaeology & History Society, 1988.

Harwood, Elaine, "The New River", Report by English Heritage, August 1989.

Rooke, P.E. (ed.), "Theobalds through the Centuries", October 1980.

Note

The former New River pumping station known as the Castle, Green Lanes, Stoke Newington, built in 1856, is now an indoor climbing centre and the west reservoir has become a facility where adults and children learn to sail. In 1995 Nicholas Grimshaw & Partners were responsible for the imaginative concept and the climbing centre's design.

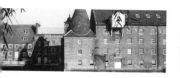

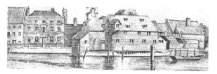

2. ENVIRONMENTALLY FRIENDLY IN THE EIGHTEENTH CENTURY

The relatively secluded site of Three Mills at Bromley-by-Bow has, over the years, experienced many changes and has also been a place where innovative processes were born. For example Dr Chaim Weizmann, who became the first President of Israel in 1948, came to work at Three Mills during the Great War. Having developed the process for producing acetone in bulk, he had been invited to set up a manufacturing process for the large-scale production of the material – at the time, urgently needed for making explosives in support of the war effort. However, there are many other interesting stories attached to this quite extraordinary site that is now situated within a conservation area at the foot of the Lea Valley; and it is probable that, as research continues, there will be more to come.

The history of the site goes back a long way. In the Domesday Survey of 1086 it is recorded that in the Manors of East and West Ham there were eight mills, formerly nine. Currently, it is not possible to say with absolute certainty that any of these were

The restored eighteenth-century House Mill at Bromley-by-Bow. Note the water channel below the mill to allow the water on the incoming tide to pass underneath. Before the tide could turn, sluice gates would be lowered to pen the water behind the four mill wheels. By raising one or more of the gates the miller could operate the mill for between twelve and sixteen hours per day. This type of mill is called a 'tide mill'.

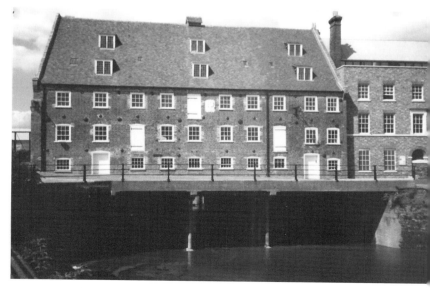

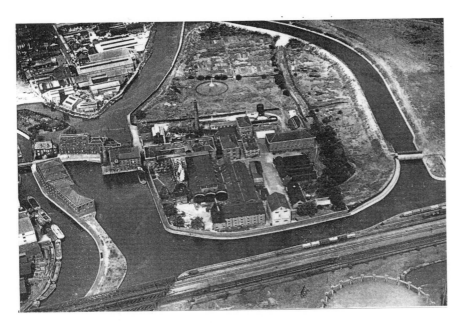

situated on the present-day site of Three Mills. However, until further evidence is uncovered to either confirm or deny this, it might be fair to conclude that one or more of the mills referred to in the Domesday Survey probably did occupy the site. Today only two mills remain from a different period: the House Mill built by the second Daniel Bisson in 1776 and the Clock Mill erected by Philip Medcalf in 1817. The clock tower, bell and clock face of the latter building are from an earlier mill of circa 1750, as are the two drying kiln towers.

An aerial view of Three Mills showing the island and various waterway channels surrounding the site (c.1938).

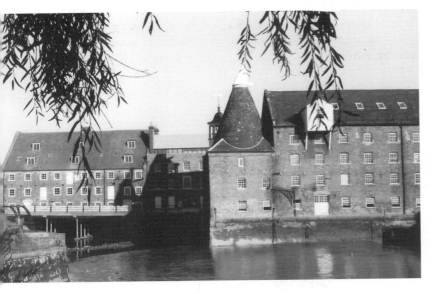

The scene at Three Mills today. To the left of the picture is the restored eighteenth-century House Mill and to the right is the early nineteenth-century Clock Mill (both are tide mills). The clock and the two drying kiln towers (once there were six) are from an earlier mill.

An "exploded" line drawing of the House Mill, showing the central water channel and four water wheels, drawn by Dr Denis Smith.

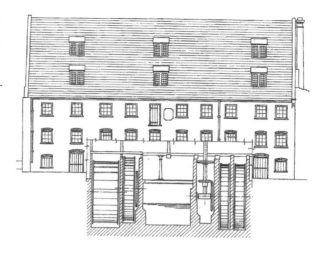

Both the House Mill and the Clock Mill were of the tidal type and employed undershot wheels, four in the former and three in the latter. Advantage was taken of the tidal properties of the lower reaches of the River Lea, fed from the River Thames, when the energy from the incoming tide was stored and used to power the mills. The high tide was allowed to flow uninhibited through a central channel below the House Mill and around fifty-seven acres of water (the surface area) was penned in the channels behind the mill to achieve the necessary force to sustain prolonged operation. When the tide began to ebb, individual sluice gates could be opened, in a controlled way, behind each water wheel, in both the House and Clock Mills, allowing the returning current to create the power to drive the grinding machinery and to operate the grain hoists. In 1938 it was calculated that, by using this system of stored energy, both mills could operate for periods of between six to eight hours on each tide thereby achieving twelve to sixteen hours working a day.

A nineteenth-century map of Essex "sewers" showing the various water channels adjacent to Three Mills. The term "sewer" was often used to mean an uncovered water channel and was not what we would think of as a sewer today.

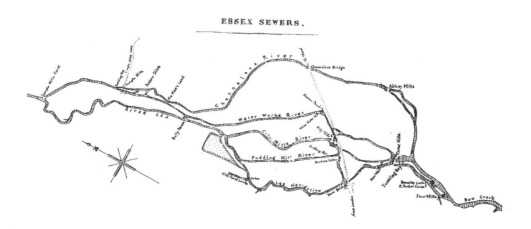

ESSEX SEWERS.

Research carried out by Dr Keith Fairclough and Mr Brian Strong of the River Lea Tidal Mill Trust would suggest that the early mills on the site were in the possession of the Abbey of Stratford Langthorne (founded in 1134–1135 by William de Montfichet), until Dissolution of the Monasteries occurred in 1538 under King Henry VIII. According to Dr Fairclough:

> for centuries before 1728 the Three Mills had been an important corn mill supplying raw materials for the Stratford and London bakers. The only exception to this pattern was that during the reign of Elisabeth I part of the facilities were used for brief periods to produce oil or gunpowder and that in the eighteenth century part of the facilities were used in the preparation of cloth.

As I have already suggested, there are many interesting stories that can be written on the subject of Three Mills; but the one that I should like to feature here is about what might be termed an eighteenth-century environmentally friendly production system that was both efficient and profitable.

When Peter Lefevre, the son of a Huguenot immigrant, purchased Three Mills and leased the nearby St Thomas Mills in 1728 the activities of the site were about to change dramatically. Lefevre, who was a baker and a mealman, had wanted to continue flour production at the mills. However, in less than a decade, Lefevre and his partners had decided to diversify their interests by setting up a brewing, distilling and pig-breeding business. Dr Fairclough has used the insurance records of the Lefevre business and the companies that followed, between the mid eighteenth and early nineteenth centuries, to estimate the size of the operation, which he concluded… *was extremely large*. In making this deduction, Dr Fairclough had taken insurance information that had been used to calculate the premiums paid on a known design of Arkwright cotton mill and compared this to the amount paid by Lefevre.

An early nineteenth-century drawing of the Three Mills area, showing the House Mill, the Clock Mill and a windmill. The windmill was destroyed by fire but the name 'Three Mills' has obviously survived.

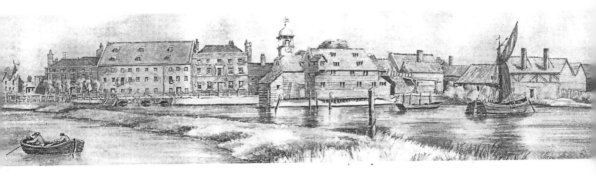

For the day, the Three Mills industries of brewing, distilling and pig breeding appear to have formed a highly successful integrated production system that took place on a site of around fifteen acres. The milling process produced flour for the bakeries of London and also prepared grain for the production of malt, beer and spirit. Waste material from these processes was fed to pigs and in turn these animals became bacon. While our eighteenth-century ancestors seemed to be well aware of the efficiency of the food-processing method they had devised, they had probably not appreciated that they had also created what we would recognise today as a basic flow-line production system – grain in – flour, brewing material, distilling material and bacon out. The choice of pigs to devour the waste from the production processes, rather than other domestic animals, meant that their meat could be cured as bacon, which gave it a much longer shelf life over un-cured meat. This had the added advantage of allowing the product to be sold cheaply in relatively small quantities. In the days before refrigeration, bacon could provide a good source of protein to supplement the diet of the less well off.

In their business partnership, Peter Lefevre and his nephew John would appear to have maintained their enterprise on a sound commercial footing through obtaining contracts to supply large quantities of bacon to the Royal Navy. Their business at Three Mills also had the advantage of allowing transport costs to the Navy storehouses to be kept to a minimum. The Royal Navy Victualling Yards were at Deptford, a short distance up the Thames from the mouth of the River Lea so it would have been quite a simple matter to move the product by water.

Lefevre was one of the larger London distillers and this side of his business was also profitable. Much of the raw alcohol produced at Three Mills was sold on to other distillers in the capital for the production of gin and other spirits. In the early part of the eighteenth century, gin was a popular drink among the working classes and with Lefevre's distilling and brewing capacity he had the ability to satisfy both the spirit and beer markets.

Our early ancestors, who made the decision to locate their milling complex on the tidal section of the lower River Lea, would appear to have been blessed with considerable planning foresight. Not only did the waterway provide power to turn the mills but it also allowed bulk quantities of grain to be brought right up to the site for easy unloading. And of course, the river provided a plentiful supply of water for the brewing and distilling processes.

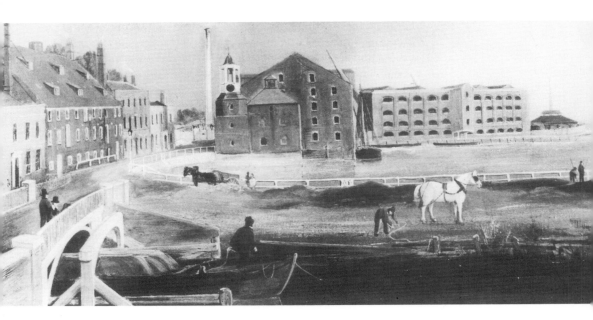

When Lefevre set up his environmentally friendly business, the thought of establishing a facility to reduce Britain's carbon footprint would never have entered his mind. It is only now, in the twenty-first century, that we are beginning to understand the mechanisms that are thought to be responsible for the conditions that have created global warming. However, it is probably fair to say that there is not yet unanimity of opinion among scientists.

A painting by I.M. Huggins of Three Mills c.1840 showing a building to the left of the House Mill and another to the right of the miller's house. Note that the two drying kilns, that are part of the Clock Mill today, are missing. It is thought that the building to the right of the Clock Mill is a type of drying kiln.

The Industrial Revolution had begun in Britain towards the end of the eighteenth century when steam power, to work the cotton looms and other factory processes, began to replace the sometimes unreliable driving force of water. Now coal, to produce the vast quantities of steam required by industry was mined and burned by the ton, creating enormous emissions of polluting smoke and chemicals and the process of global warming began, although the condition at the time was not appreciated.

With the expansion of the railway network towards the middle of the nineteenth century, it became relatively easy to move large quantities of coal from the mines located in the midlands and the north of the country to the rapidly expanding industries of the south. The burning of fossil fuels, as one might expect, created an increase in the pollution of the environment on a dramatic scale. Not only was the discharge of smoke from factory chimneys a problem, but factory owners began dumping vast amounts of industrial waste on open land, in rivers and in the sea.

As consumerism took hold in the twentieth century, with the increasing public appetite for cheap manufactured goods, countries around the world became industrialised to meet demand. The result of this manufacturing boom significantly contributed to the effect which has now become known as global warming. Now scientists and world leaders are trying to find different environmentally friendly ways to manufacture our goods and to grow and produce our food. This, paradoxically, is almost three hundred years after Lefevre had, almost by accident, stumbled upon an environmentally friendly method of food and drink production.

REFERENCES

Fairclough, Keith, "The Three Mills Distillery in the Georgian Era", River Lea Tidal Mill Trust Ltd.

Fairclough, Keith, "Philip Metcalfe (1733–1818) The MP and Industrialist who Built the Clock Mill", River Lea Tidal Mill Trust Ltd.

Fairclough, Keith, "Owners of the Three Mills (1539–1728")", River Lea Tidal Mill Trust Ltd.

Fairclough, Keith, "The Lefevre Family and Distilling Along the Lower Lea", River Lea Tidal Mill Trust Ltd.

Fairclough, Keith and Strong, Brian, "The Bisson Family of Three Mills", River Lea Tidal Mill Trust Ltd.

Note

The House Mill at Three Mills, Bromley-by-Bow, is open every Sunday (2pm–4pm) between May and October. Further information can be obtained by telephoning: 0208 980 4626.

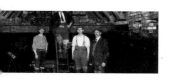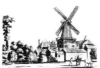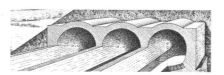

3. THE MAN WHO DID LONDON'S DIRTY WORK

Joseph William Bazalgette (later Sir Joseph), not to be confused with his father who was also Joseph William Bazalgette, a Commander in the Royal Navy, was born at Enfield, Middlesex, on 28 March 1819. The precise place of his birth was initially unknown, but by using historic maps, parish records and completing much more detective work, his birthplace was traced to a Georgian farmhouse that once stood towards the top of Clay Hill, Enfield a short distance below the Fallow Buck public house.

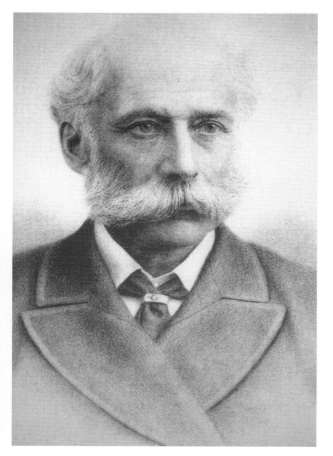

Sir Joseph Bazalgette (1819–1891).

After an education at private schools, Bazalgette became a pupil of Sir John Benjamin MacNeill in 1836, the same year in which he joined the Institution of Civil Engineers. MacNeill had begun his career under the famous civil engineer Thomas Telford and became one of his deputies. Telford clearly had a high regard for MacNeill: after his death in 1834 it was discovered that he had remembered him in his will.

Bazalgette's early experience of carrying out work on a drainage and reclamation project in the north of Ireland, and his involvement in other tasks as a pupil of MacNeill, helped shape what was to become a highly distinguished career in civil engineering. By 1842 he had set up at Westminster as a consulting engineer, being mainly engaged on railway work.

By the mid nineteenth century there had been a number of serious cholera outbreaks, but the epidemics of 1849 and 1854 alone had claimed the lives of almost forty-thousand people. While poor sanitation and lack of clean supplies of drinking water were thought to be the main causes of the problem, there were other contributory factors like the random dumping of household waste in the streets, which, over the years, had gone unchecked.

When the Romans built Londinium, their settlement by the Thames, in about AD 50, the river and its tributaries would have been clear and unpolluted. Since that time, a gradual increase and then a rapid expansion in the population and their dwellings had taken place, putting considerable pressure on nature's resources, land and water. For example, in the first fifty years of the nineteenth century, the number of people living in the capital had quadrupled. The Metropolis Management Act of 1855 defined London as having a population of almost 4,000,000 inhabitants living in 500,000 houses, which covered an area of 117 square miles. Apart from the increased levels of pollution created by such a large population, with their human waste leaching into rivers and streams, there was also the added problem of industrial effluent discharge as a growing number of factories were setting up in London. Over the years little had been done to deal with these mounting difficulties and the mere fact that the ground had been covered with buildings and roads meant that there was hardly any natural space to soak up surface rainwater. During wet weather, rain would mix with the untreated sewage from cesspools and other areas causing extra run-off into the already polluted rivers and streams. This, in turn, caused flooding of the noxious soup on to streets, walkways and into cellars, the results of which would not have been particularly pleasant for residents living in these areas or nearby.

In 1849 Bazalgette became a member of the Metropolitan Commission of Sewers. Appointments to this body were government nominations. The new organisation had been set up in the previous year to replace the eight different district bodies that had been responsible for the drainage of London. Previously, little thought had been given to a method of uniform drainage for the capital and as a consequence the system was completely outdated and extremely inefficient. Because there had not been one coordinating body charged with design and development, there were considerable differences of size, shape and fall of the sewers at the district boundaries, with larger sewers discharging into smaller ones and egg-shaped sewers with narrow parts uppermost coupled to similar sewers built in reverse. The result in times of heavy usage was effluent back up (surcharge) and blockage.

Workmen in the Fleet sewer
(the old River Fleet, a lost
London river) c.1900.

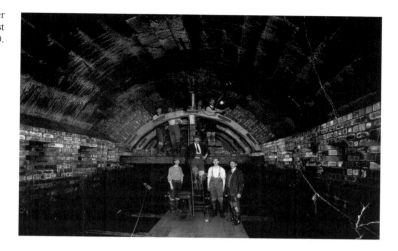

Up until 1815 it was illegal to discharge sewage or other noxious
material into the sewers as it had been deemed they should only be
used to carry surface water. At the time, cesspools were considered
to be the only place appropriate for depositing household sewage.
Incidentally, the term "sewer" has not always meant a brick-lined
tunnel to take away household effluent. Various rivers and streams,
that took away surface water, were often referred to as sewers. As
cesspools were the only places where household effluent could
effectively be stored, it is therefore obvious that these pits would
quickly fill up. Removing the sewage from these smelly receptacles
was the unpleasant job of the "night men" who took the waste away
from the resident's homes, but were not always over particular
where they dumped the unhygienic contents.

However, with London's dramatic increase in population it is clear
that cesspools were unable to cope with the mounting levels of
waste. Also, the inadequate system of disposing of the effluent had
not been helped by the introduction of the water closet into some
of London's more affluent homes in the late eighteenth century.
This had increased loading on the antiquated cesspool system as
the flushing toilet gained popularity. These pressures appear to have
been temporally addressed when the law, restricting the discharge
of sewerage, was either deliberately relaxed, or perhaps a blind eye
was turned by the authorities in an effort to save money. It was not
until 1847 that an act was passed which made it compulsory to
drain household waste into London's sewers. Within six years,
thirty-thousand cesspools had been abolished as the effluent was
directed into a modified, but not redesigned, sewerage system. Now
surface water and raw sewage combined to be discharged directly

into the River Thames. In many instances the outflows of sewage were close to where the private water companies and ordinary Londoners took their supplies.

Although Joseph Bazalgette had been appointed a member of the Metropolitan Commission of Sewers in 1849 and in the years that followed several plans were submitted to the Commission for improving London's sewer system, none were implemented. However, in 1854 Bazalgette was directed to "prepare a scheme of intercepting sewers, intended to effect the improved Main Drainage of London, and Mr Haywood was associated with him for the northern portion". In February that year, the talented civil engineer Sir William Cubitt reported, seemingly enthusiastically, that:

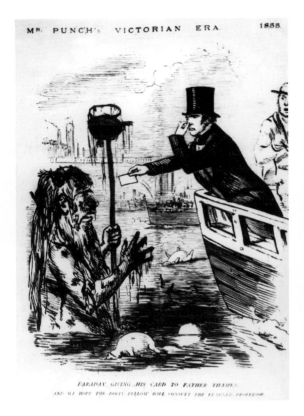

MR. PUNCH'S VICTORIAN ERA. 1855.

FARADAY GIVING HIS CARD TO FATHER THAMES
AND WE HOPE THE DIRTY FELLOW WILL CONSULT THE LEARNED PROFESSOR.

> after a very careful examination of the reports and plans, and the elaborate set of sections and details which they [Messrs, Bazalgette and Haywood] have produced, together with the estimate founded thereon, that the whole are worthy of every attention as regards the capacities and inclinations of the various intercepting drains, in relation to the quantities of water they have to carry and discharge.

Even though Cubitt appears to have suggested that Bazalgette and Haywood's plan should be considered seriously, the Commission still took no action.

A Punch cartoon depicting the celebrated electrical engineer Michael Faraday meeting Old Father Thames at the time of the 'Great Stink'. Faraday is holding a slip of litmus paper in his hand and it was these that he used to test the purity of Thames water.

Between 1848 and 1855 the Metropolitan Commission of Sewers had been reconstituted six times with successive new appointments. This made it almost impossible for the body to implement any worthwhile schemes of sufficient magnitude to alleviate the growing sewerage problems. They were also not in a strong position to tackle the other major issue, the unsatisfactory state of the highly polluted River Thames, which appears to have become London's main sewer. The water companies which took their supplies from the Thames were coming under increasing pressure as concern for the health of the general public intensified. In London, the total deaths from cholera alone, in 1854, amounted to almost twenty thousand. Although Bazalgette had been appointment Chief Engineer of the fifth and sixth Commissions, his early plans for solving London's drainage problems remained frustrated.

As mentioned earlier, the removal of 30,000 cesspools from the capital had caused high levels of raw sewage to enter the Thames, sometimes close to where water companies were extracting drinking water. Now the pollution of the river had become so bad that in 1855 an act was passed "to prevent all sewage from the Metropolis flowing into the Thames". Of course, politicians sitting comfortably in Parliament and passing an act is one thing; making such a scheme happen and then monitoring its progress is another.

In 1856, under a further act of Parliament, the Metropolitan Board of Works was set up, superseding the Metropolitan Commission of Sewers. This body was the first serious attempt to bring about a system of local self-government by dividing the capital into thirty-nine districts. The City of London and the largest parishes, like Lambeth and Marylebone, formed separate districts, while the smaller parishes were amalgamated into further individual districts of manageable size. Bazalgette was appointed Chief Engineer to this new body and instructed to prepare plans for the drainage of London. This he duly did and the scheme was approved by the Board. However, Her Majesty's First Commissioner of Works had the power of veto and Bazalgette's plan was frustratingly delayed. After much complicated negotiation and discussion, his recommendations were eventually adopted and work began on the scheme in 1859.

It is possible that Members of Parliament may, out of self-interest, have put pressure on those delaying progress: in the summer of 1858, when temperatures in the metropolis exceeded ninety degrees Fahrenheit, raw sewerage was brought up the Thames to Westminster on the incoming tide. It is reported that the disgusting smell from the highly polluted river became so unbearable for the finer sensitivities of some of the sitting members that the windows and doors of the Houses of Parliament had to be covered with curtains soaked in chloride of lime to try to overcome the dreadful stench. The episode became known as the "Great Stink" and it may have been this "effluent lobby of parliament" that created the necessary political will that gave Bazalgette the final authority to begin work on his scheme.

Bazalgette's grand plan was to construct a sewerage system which, as far as possible, would rely upon gravity and surface water to ensure that effluent was kept flowing. He also planned to divert the waste away from outlets which fed directly into the Thames near the centre of London, to a place some fourteen miles below London Bridge. He had calculated that by discharging at this distance there would be little chance of the sewage being brought back to the metropolis by the turning tide.

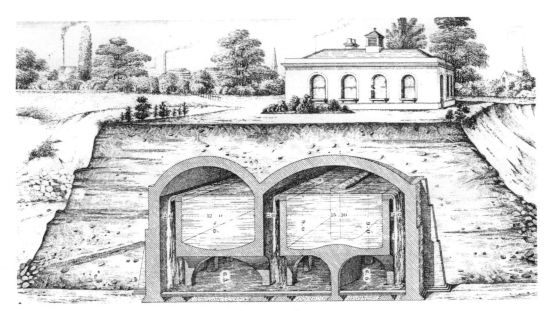

A drawing showing a section of the overflow chamber at the junction of the northern, high and middle level sewers.

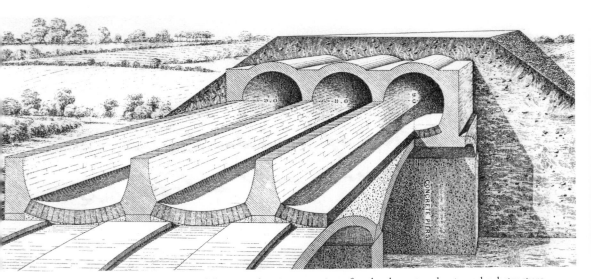

A drawing of the Northern Outfall Sewer showing a section of embankment, culverts and substructure.

A nineteenth-century engraving of the Abbey Mills Pumping Station. Apart from the twin chimneys being demolished in 1941 to make the site a less obvious target for German bombers, the building still retains many of its original features including the bases of the now demolished chimneys.

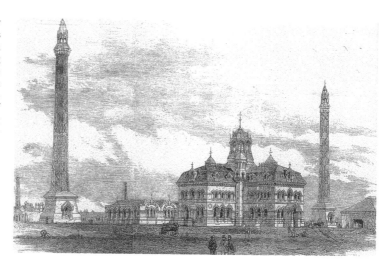

In surveying the existing sewerage system, Bazalgette soon discovered it was not possible, for reasons already outlined, to use the existing network of water channels and tunnels. His ambitious plan was effectively to start from scratch by constructing three intercepting sewers (high, middle and low level) north of the River Thames running west to east, all relying on gravity and using surface water to maintain the flow. On the south side of the river the three intercepting lines (high and low level, plus the Effra Branch) all met at Deptford Creek. Here he planned to install pumps to lift the sewage eighteen feet (5.3 metres) into the Southern Outfall Sewer. From there, the waste material would be taken by gravity to Crossness on the Erith Marshes where massive steam engines would pump the waste into storage tanks, later to be discharged into the Thames on the ebb tide. The choice of the Erith Marshes took into account Bazalgette's calculation that sewage would not be returned to the capital on the incoming tide if the discharged was made fourteen miles below London Bridge.

The plan for West Ham, situated on the north side of the Thames and on the Essex side of the River Lea, was to build a pumping station at Abbey Mills to lift the effluent around forty feet (12 metres) from the low level sewer to feed the Northern Outfall Sewer. Once there, under the power of gravity, the material would flow onward to Barking Creek where it would be stored in tanks to await discharge into the Thames on the ebb tide. Bazalgette's massive scheme of approximately 1,300 miles of brick-built sewers took almost sixteen years to complete and is the backbone of our sewerage system today, playing a vital part in the maintenance of London's health in the twenty-first century.

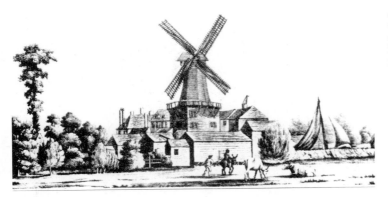

An eighteenth-century picture of the old Abbey Windmill, sited close to where Bazalgette's pumping station now stands.

Presumably in an effort to disguise its unromantic occupation from local residents, the Abbey Mills pumping station was constructed on a grand scale in the form of a cross, with a central lantern, mansard roof and dormer windows. It also included ornamental coloured brickwork, arched windows, sculptured masonry, expensive wall tiles and, on the inside, a profusion of decorative and lavishly constructed ironwork. The design of the building was the work of Bazalgette and Edmund Cooper. To finish off the construction, the architect, Charles Driver, designed two highly ornate Moorish style chimneys, each a hundred and ninety feet (58 metres) tall. These took away the exhaust from the boilers that fed four pairs of beam engines located (two in each section) within the four sections of

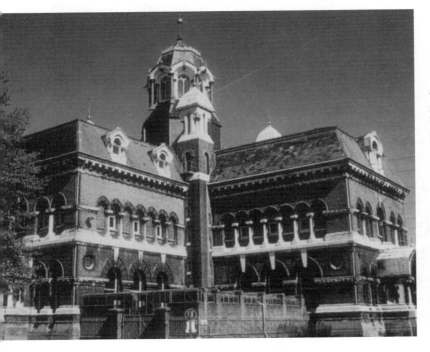

The Abbey Mills Pumping Station, Stratford, London, built c.1868. Because of its ornate design, the building became known as the "Cathedral of Sewage". Originally, beam engines were employed to lift the lower-level sewage into the Northern Outfall Sewer (constructed between 1860 and 1865) where the effluent mixed with surface water before being discharge into the River Thames at Barking. Later improvements to the system saw the separation from the effluent of solids, which were taken out to sea in "gravy boats" for dumping.

An engraving showing the inside of the Abbey Mills Pumping Station with its profusion of intricate Victorian ironwork. Although the pumping station is now only used in emergencies in cases of severe flooding, the ironwork remains in all its Victorian glory.

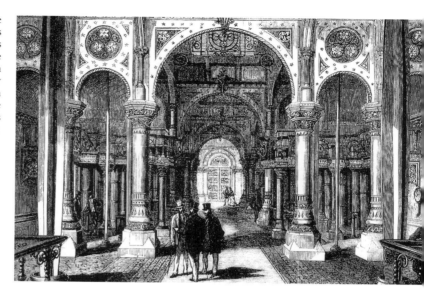

The base of one of Bazalgette's massive chimneys that remain in the grounds of Abbey Mills Pumping Station.

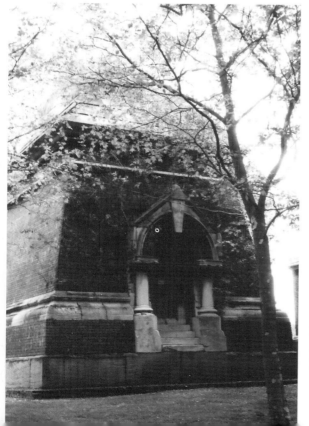

the cruciform shape. The overall effect of the masonry was so exquisite and flamboyant that the building was nicknamed the "Cathedral of Sewage" and, on occasion, also referred to as "a mosque in the marshes".

The Abbey Mills pumping station had its beam engines removed in 1933 when powerful electric pumps were installed to take over the work. Although the Abbey Mills pumping station still stands, sadly the chimneys were demolished by the authorities after bombs damaged some of the site's low-level buildings in 1941. At the time, it was thought that the chimneys provided the German aircrews with a highly visible landmark to target the London Docks. (One would have thought that enemy aircraft flying across the North Sea and making landfall in Britain would have used the much larger Thames to navigate their route to the Docks.) However, the bases of the chimneys still remain and are fine examples of architecture of the period.

Recently, English Heritage listed the main building Grade II* after a programme of restoration work was carried out in conjunction with Thames Water. The facility, now known as the "A" Station, was relegated to standby status in 1997 and deals with pumping storm water at times of emergency, thereby being available to protect large areas of London from flooding. A modern state-of-the-art pumping station, to a design developed by Thames Water engineers, has been built nearby and was commissioned in 1997. This facility is one of the largest sewage pumping stations in the world, serving over one million people in London and other low-lying areas north of the Thames. Instead of discharging solids into the lower reaches of the Thames or dumping at sea, a £165 million sludge incineration plant was opened at Beckton (near Barking Creek) in 1998 and a sludge-powered generator was commissioned at Crossness. These eco-friendly establishments can generate sufficient electricity to run the plants and supply surplus power to the national grid.

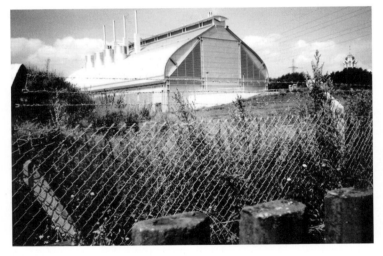

The modern state-of-the-art pumping station at Abbey Mills, to a design developed by Thames Water engineers and commissioned in 1997. This facility is one of the largest sewage pumping stations in the world, serving over one million people in London and other low-lying areas north of the Thames.

Fortunately, in recent years, there has been increased interest in the preservation of industrial buildings. Abbey Mills stands as a memorial to Victorian engineering ingenuity, in an area of Stratford that is fast regenerating, driven by the many infrastructure developments surrounding the forthcoming Olympic and Paralympic Games. Before his death in March 1891, Bazalgette would have been entitled to look back on his remarkable career with pride. Together with an army of workmen, craftsmen and skilled engineers, he had restored the health of London's population and his legacy is still being enjoyed today – as no doubt it will be by future generations.

REFERENCES

Bazalgette, Joseph William, "On the Main Drainage of London and the Interception of the Sewage from the River Thames", Minutes of Proceedings of the Institution of Civil Engineers, 14 March 1865, Volume 24, 1864–1865.

Bazalgette, Joseph William, "Address of Sir J.W. Bazalgette, President", Minutes of Proceedings of the Institution of Civil Engineers, 8 January 1884.

Clayton, Anthony, *Subterranean City Beneath the Streets of London*, Historical Publications, 2000.

Lee, Sidney (ed.), *Dictionary of National Biography*, Volume XXII, Smith Elder & Co., London, 1909.

Lee, Sidney (ed.), *Dictionary of National Biography*, Volume XXIL, Smith Elder & Co., London, 1909.

Lewis, Jim, *London's Lea Valley – Britain's Best Kept Secret*, Phillimore & Company Ltd., Chichester, 1999.

Lewis, Jim, *East Ham and West Ham Past*, Historical Publications Ltd., London, 2004.

Note

At the time of writing, Thames Water has two major schemes, both at the planning and consultation stage, to deal with the recurring problem of untreated effluent being discharged into London's river systems during times of heavy rainfall. Over the years, as the population of London has grown and virgin land has increasingly disappeared under buildings and roads (not to mention car-owning residents paving over their front gardens to provide off-road parking for one or more cars), the absorption of water into the ground during storms has been considerably curtailed. At such times, surface water has no place to go but into the roadside drains, which were never designed to take the increased volumes, and inevitably the system becomes overloaded, causing flooding. At such times, Thames Water has no option but to discharge the overcapacity into the Channelsea River at Stratford, Barking Creek and also into the Thames. Unfortunately, due to Bazalgette's design of the London sewerage system, which uses surface water (rainfall) as a flushing agent, household effluent is discharged along with the surface water at the various outlet points.

The first scheme is to develop a four-mile spur tunnel (Lee Tunnel) from Abbey Mills Pumping Station to Beckton Sewage Treatment Works (STW). This will relieve pressure, in time of storms, on the Northern Outfall Sewer. Before being transferred to the tunnel for storage, the effluent will be passed through screens to remove the majority of the sewage solids. After the storm has passed, the tunnel will be pumped out and the effluent will be treated at Beckton. The Lee Tunnel route will follow the line of the Northern Outfall Sewer that is located under the "Greenway". Tunnelling techniques, not

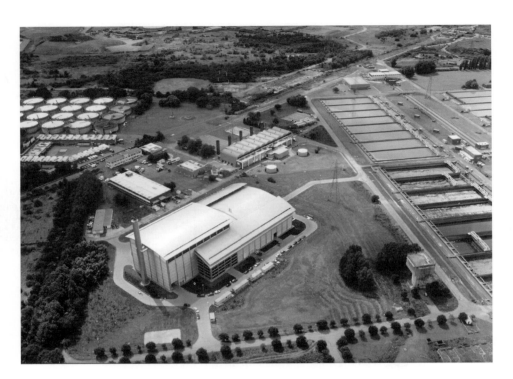

An aerial view of the modern Beckton sewage treatment plant.

too dissimilar to those used during the recent boring of the under Channel rail link, will be employed at a depth of between fifty-five and seventy metres. Removal of the tunnel spoil, mainly a mixture of wet chalk, will be by conveyor at the Beckton STW end and from there by barge to its final destination.

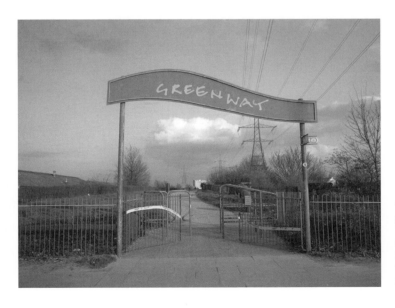

The Greenway which runs along the line of Bazalgette's 150-year-old Northern Outfall Sewer. This has provided Londoners with a pleasant walking and cycling route for many years.

The route of the proposed Thames Water Tideway Tunnel, planned to provide a solution to London's mounting storm-water problems.

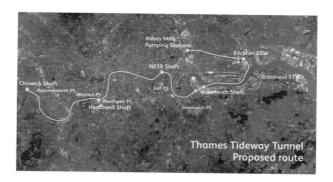

The second scheme is to build the Tideway Tunnel which will follow the route of the River Thames from a point just north of Wandsworth to its termination at Beckton STW. Again, after the storm has passed the tunnel will be pumped out and the effluent treated. It is estimated that this tunnel will pick up approximately 98 percent of the combined sewers' output that would normally have had to be discharged into the River Thames at times of heavy rainfall.

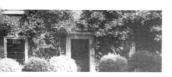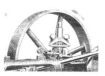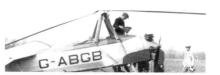

4. THE LEA VALLEY EXPERIENCE – A SHOWCASE PROJECT IN PROGRESS

I could not write this new series of books on London's Lea Valley without recording my sincere admiration for a group of enthusiastic volunteers who have worked tirelessly for over fourteen years to establish an interpretation centre, the Lea Valley Experience, to showcase a host of world industrial firsts and to tell the many unique stories about the region. At the time of writing, the author cannot be confident that sufficient funding will be made available for the whole project to succeed. If it does, however, the Lea Valley will have a major educational and tourist attraction in time for the 2012 Olympics, one that could rival Ironbridge Gorge in Shropshire and Beamish in County Durham.

The Low Hall Pump House, a Grade II Victorian building constructed in 1885.

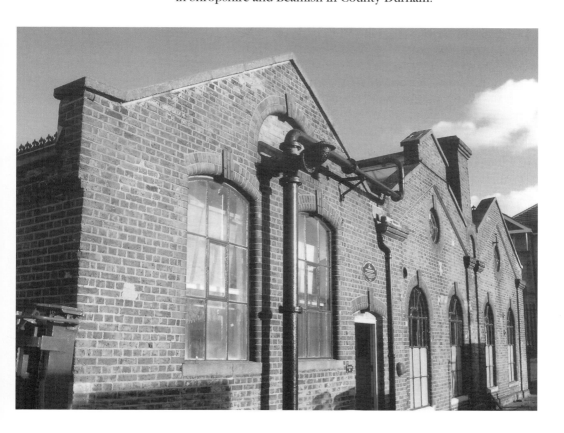

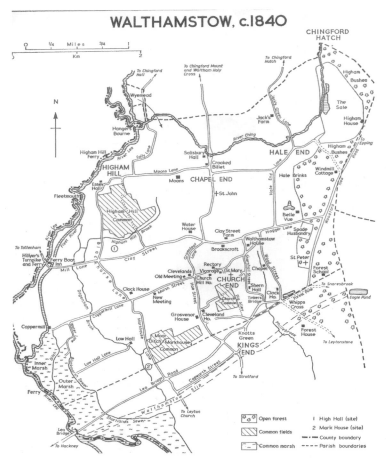

WALTHAMSTOW, c.1840

A Walthamstow map of c.1840 showing the site of Low Hall, positioned towards the bottom left-hand corner and adjacent to Dagenham Brook. The map is reproduced with permission of the editor of *The Victoria History of the County of Essex, Vol. VI*.

The project is currently located in a Grade II listed former Victorian sewage-pumping station in an area of Waltham Forest known as Low Hall that borders Walthamstow Marsh. Traditionally, local authorities have used such low-lying areas to locate their less-attractive facilities away from public gaze and sometimes from sensitive noses. Nevertheless, the varied history of the site, which goes back centuries, is on a par with those that have been publicly acclaimed national treasures. While it is important to tell the stories of kings, queens, generals and stately homes, these should be balanced against the interpretation of industrial history and civil engineering, the behind-the-scenes driving force that has defined the way we have developed and live today. If we neglect to do this, we shall fail to understand the bigger historical picture.

Ownership of the land now known as Low Hall can be traced back to Anglo-Saxon times, although early records of ownership are

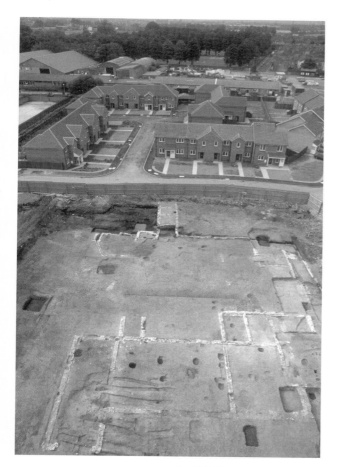

Aerial view of the excavations of Low Hall Manor carried out by the Museum of London Archaeology Services (MOLAS) that discovered remains of a high-status moated manor house with evidence of later extensions and alterations.

sketchy and require a degree of interpretation. However, a more comprehensive picture emerges after the Norman Conquest, thanks to William the Conqueror and the Domesday Survey of 1086. In a publication of this type, it would not be appropriate to list every owner of the Low Hall lands up to recent times; we shall therefore begin with the background to Walthamstow Local Board's acquisition of the land.

Charles Burrell had leased the land at Low Hall, then comprising of around 225 acres, from Samuel Bosanquet in 1843. The Bosanquet family were successful merchants of Huguenot descent, who had, like many of their countrymen, fled France to escape religious persecution. The family became British subjects in 1698 and in 1741 they bought the land at Low Hall. In 1877 the fourth named Samuel Bosanquet, the last Lord of the Manor, sold the grounds and buildings at Low Hall for £25,300 to the Walthamstow Local Board. However, the family appear to have held a vested interest in the site until 1926. This was because Bosanquet had negotiated the right to hold Manor Courts in the farm house. Readers of a certain age may remember the popular television newscaster Reginald Bosanquet, a descendant of the family.

A BRIEF HISTORY OF LOW HALL STRUCTURES AND THE EXCAVATIONS BY THE MUSEUM OF LONDON IN 1997

Archaeology Services (MOLAS) discovered the remains of a high-status moated manor house with evidence of later extensions and alterations. Archaeologists have concluded that wood recovered from the dig had once formed part of a base frame, which helped support a drawbridge crossing the moat. Dendrochronology (the science of dating by the examination of tree rings) has dated the wood to the summer of 1344 and it is thought that the original manor house would have been contemporary with this date. Further discoveries from the dig have revealed that the original moated manor house

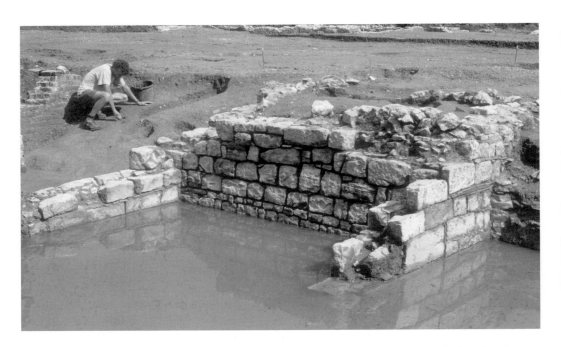

was levelled sometime during the seventeenth century when buildings of a lesser status were erected. During the eighteenth and nineteenth centuries the main building seems to have gone through a change of use, eventually becoming a farmhouse. During the Second World War (1939–1945), on the morning of 18 August 1944, a German V1 flying bomb did what time had failed to do and removed the last standing piece of Low Hall heritage. This was exactly six hundred years after the building of the medieval manor house in 1344. Artefacts recovered from the dig included a large piece of the flying bomb.

The modified medieval bridge abutment exposed during the 1997 excavations of Low Hall Manor by Museum of London Archaeology Services (MOLAS). It is thought that the moat would have been filled with water from the nearby Dagenham Brook via a system of sluices.

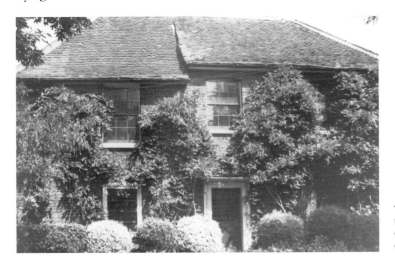

The farmhouse at Low Hall that was destroyed by a German V1 flying bomb (Doodlebug) in August 1944.

The only known surviving picture of outbuildings and working animals at Low Hall Farm.

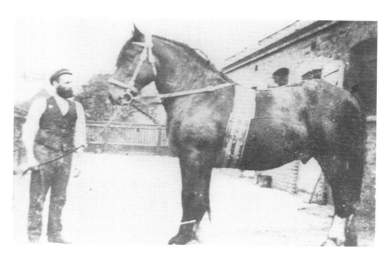

LOW HALL'S PROGRESS FROM THE LATE NINETEENTH CENTURY

The purchase of land at Low Hall in 1877, by the Walthamstow Local Board, was to assist with the growing problem of treating and disposing of sewage and also to improve drainage. With the coming of the railways towards the middle of the nineteenth century the population of Walthamstow had dramatically increased from 7,137 in 1861 to 22,531 in 1881, and by the turn of the century had expanded over fourfold to 96,720. No doubt the board members were mindful of the cholera and typhoid epidemics of the mid nineteenth century that had accounted for the deaths of thousands of Londoners. Interestingly, it was a Lea Valley man born in Enfield, Sir Joseph Bazalgette, who designed and oversaw the construction of the London sewerage system that helped to eradicate these diseases.

Before Bazalgette's massive civil-engineering scheme had taken place, the central areas of London had to rely mainly on a system of cesspits to store the raw sewage. These had to be emptied by the "night men" and the effluent disposed of, not always hygienically. Many of the cesspits overflowed and effluent also leached through the ground into the rivers, streams and also the aquifer. Unfortunately, outer-lying London districts like Walthamstow, probably because of financial constraints, had not been connected to the new system of sewers and still relied heavily on cesspits and other crude methods of sewage disposal.

By 1880, work had begun on the construction of a simple sewage treatment plant on the north side of Low Hall, consisting mainly of filter beds and sludge tanks. After chemical treatment, the solids were dried and pressed before being taken away to be spread on farmland; but it is known that solids were often spread on fields without too much processing. While the administration of Low Hall Sewerage Farm, as it became known, was under the control of a Council committee, the operation of the plant had been leased to a private contractor. As might be imagined the operation was not a success as complaints from local residents and neighbouring authorities began to increase due to the pollution of watercourses and also because of unpleasant smells that became particularly pungent during periods of hot weather.

In 1884, pressured by the level of complaint, the Council terminated the contractor's lease of Low Hall Sewerage Farm and took over the running of the works. The following year, under the supervision of George Benstall Jerram, the Council's surveyor and engineer, a complete redevelopment of the site took place. Eli Wilson, a local builder, was given the job of constructing a two-bayed engine house and Tangye Ltd. of Birmingham was approached to tender for the work of supplying and installing steam pumps and boilers. The choice of the Tangye brothers' company is interesting as they were the manufacturers of the powerful hydraulic jacks that eventually, to the great relief of Isambard Kingdom Brunel, launched his massive steamship the *Great Eastern*, from its construction site on the Isle of Dogs in 1858. The event provoked the now-famous saying "Tangye launched the *Great Eastern* and the *Great Eastern* launched Tangye".

The Lea Valley Experience project plans to tell the story of Brunel and his connections with the Lea Valley through his association with the Thames Iron Works, once located on the east bank of the River Lea where the waterway meets the Thames. What a

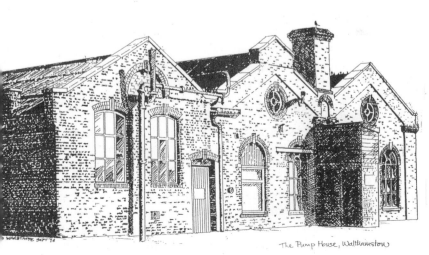

The Pump House, Walthamstow

A drawing of the Low Hall Pump House, by David Wagstaff, as it looked in September 1976.

An engraving of one of the Pump House engines, manufactured by Marshall, Sons & Co. Ltd., Gainsborough, Lincolnshire. Volunteers of the Friends of the Pump House have restored this engine to working order.

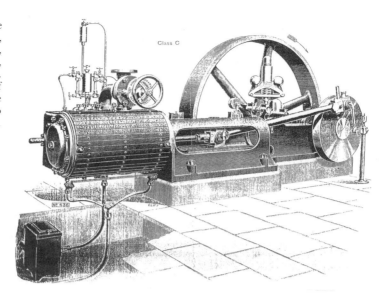

coincidence that the heritage of the Lea Valley Experience project shares a common supplier with the great Victorian engineer!

Although the new sewage works was an improvement over what had formerly existed, the arrangements were not ideal and would certainly not solve the long-term needs of an increasing population. Moreover, drainage was becoming an increasing problem as discharges from the works were polluting the local watercourses. Complaints were again received from adjacent local authorities and Walthamstow Council had little choice but to update the sewage works once more. In March 1896, the Council accepted the estimate of Marshall, Sons & Co. Ltd. of Gainsborough to supply and install a pair of coupled horizontal steam engines and a Cornish boiler. The work was completed by May the following year along with alterations to the engine house with the addition of a third bay and by raising the boiler house chimney to improve draught for the boiler furnace. These solutions were to prove highly effective in the processing of sewage for many years.

DEALING WITH HOUSEHOLD AND OTHER WASTE

In 1905, to deal with the problems of rubbish disposal, a refuse-incineration plant was erected at Low Hall, close to the Victorian pump house. Ironically, the Low Hall site that was once the grand preserve of the Lords of the Manor was now becoming a waste repository to benefit the health of ordinary people. In 1928, further changes to the works were made when connections to the London County Council sewerage system came about, allowing the Marshall engines to pump effluent directly into Bazalgette's sewers for the first time. Later, workshops were added to the site and the engines were given the extra task of powering the various machines via a system of overhead line shafting.

UPDATING AND REDUNDANCY
By the early 1960s the boilers that provided steam for the Marshall engines were becoming increasingly unreliable and were eventually condemned. The opportunity was then taken to replace the plant with a separate modern pumping system, automatic and powered by electricity. For over two decades after the engines had fallen silent, the pumping station building was used to store various items which the Council considered redundant yet wished to keep.

COMMUNITY FEARS AND INSPIRATION
In the 1970s, spurred on by rumours of the pump house being targeted for demolition, a group of likeminded enthusiasts came up with the concept of using the building and its adjacent yard to create a transport museum, with a view to highlighting the many industrial achievements that had begun life in Waltham Forest. Great ideas do not always translate into reality immediately and it was not until the early 1990s that a charitable trust was formed, and promises of a lease on the building and the yard were obtained from the local Council. Nevertheless, despite the relatively slow progress in securing all the necessary agreements, the volunteers persevered with their vision, no doubt driven by the infectious enthusiasm of Lindsay Collier, the Project Director. While the task ahead was without doubt a mammoth undertaking, things did not stand still. The volunteers grew in numbers and established a solid body of friends. One of the Marshall engines, through the exceptional skills of Melvin Mantell and his team, was coaxed back into life and can be seen working on open days. Renovation of the building, now Grade II listed, began and the museum collection increased dramatically as people from across the country donated artefacts. Themed weekends were started that became popular with the public, particularly children.

The author was particularly flattered to learn, from representatives of the Pump House Trust, that his two Lea Valley books had inspired members to look at widening the remit of the museum project from one of local focus to that of regional interpretation. The visionary concept of the Lea Valley Experience was born.

Ambitious plans have now been drawn up to create a visitor attraction that will have walk-through display galleries, temporary exhibition space, educational classrooms, community space, a street scene and a training facility. Initial funding has already come from

Four artist's impressions for the proposed Lea Valley Experience museum where it is planned to showcase the region's groundbreaking industrial achievements, many of which were world firsts.

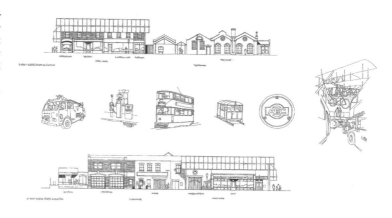

the London Borough of Waltham Forest and the Heritage Lottery Fund and a modest amount of financial backing has been received from a national retailer and support in kind from a major local business. The Trustees plan to develop the project in manageable stages, completing the opening by 2009, the year of the centenary celebrations of A.V. Roe's historic flight from Walthamstow Marsh. A replica of Roe's triplane, which has been specially built for the celebrations, will be taxied on the marsh during the festivities, which have attracted the support of a number of official bodies. Eric Verdon-Roe, A.V.'s grandson, has generously sponsored the building of the aircraft, which after the event will permanently feature in a special gallery, currently included within the plans for the Lea Valley Experience project. It is the aim of the Trustees to create a first-class tourist experience so that visitors from across the world to the 2012 Olympics can learn how the industries of the Lea Valley influenced the way we live today.

Here is a great opportunity to showcase the plethora of industrial firsts that happened locally and also to explain how the Victorians tackled problems of public health. It is therefore to be hoped that the Lea Valley Experience project will be successful in its funding applications, despite the present global financial crisis: it is important for future generations to understand the unique heritage of the region before all the stories are lost in the mists of time.

REFERENCES

Author unknown,"A Heritage Jewel for Walthamstow,The Origins of the Lea Valley Experience Museum", document published by the Trustees of the Pump House Steam & Transport Museum Trust.

Author unknown,"The Lea Valley Experience Project", News Letter published by the Trustees of the Pump House Steam & Transport Museum Trust, November 2004.

Author unknown,"Brief Summary Report on the History of the Engines and Engine House at Low Hall Depot, Low Hall Lane,Walthamstow", Prepared by Local Studies Section,Vestry House Museum, May 1994.

Blair, Ian,"Low Hall Manor,Walthamstow", *Current Archaeology*, Number 162, May 1999.

Collier, Patricia,"The Low Hall Story – An Account of Walthamstow's Past", unpublished paper.

Evans, R.J.,Archivist,Vestry House Museum, letter to D. Green, Senior Engineer, Highway Records Department of Development, London Borough of Waltham Forest, undated.

Powell,W.R. (ed.), *The Victoria History of the County of Essex, Vol.VI*, Institute of Historical Research, University of London, 1973.

Note

In previous books, the author took the opportunity to encourage others, particularly young people, to carry out research into little-known Lea Valley facts and rumours. It is hoped that this tradition will continue. Perhaps schools and other educational establishments would like to take up the challenge of researching the following Low Hall stories:

Cinder Athletics Track. As a young schoolboy in the early 1950s, the author regularly trained, with many of his athletic colleagues, on a rough-surfaced, black, oval cinder track that was sited south of the pavilion and changing rooms on the sports ground known as Low Hall Farm. For some unexplained reason, the track was of the non-standard distance (perhaps the only one in the world) of three and a bit laps to the mile. To run the mile, athletes would have to complete three laps then go a little further and finish on the top bend. This would have probably given the lap a distance of around 530 yards. At the time, running tracks were 440 yards long, so four laps equalled one mile. With the Olympics coming to the Lea Valley in 2012, this would make a great research project.

Elephant Store. Strange as it may seem, there was once a building at Low Hall to house elephants. Apparently, the circus came to Walthamstow twice a year in pre Second World War times and gave performances in the Palace Theatre that was then on the north side of High Street. The building at Low Hall, said to be timber framed, was the largest and strongest available that was near enough to the Palace to accommodate the elephants. During the Second World War the building was hit by a German incendiary bomb, which killed a number of horses that were stabled inside. In 1979 the building was demolished, after finishing its life as a storage place for road repair materials.

Isolation Hospital. In 1929, a small isolation hospital was built at Low Hall on ground to the west of Dagenham Brook. The purpose of such hospitals was to isolate smallpox patients away from the local community, to help stop this highly contagious disease spreading. In 1940 the hospital was damaged by incendiary bombs and was closed.

Alan Cobham's Flying Circus. Alan Cobham, a member of the Royal Flying Corps during the First World War, became a test pilot for the de Havilland aircraft company after the war and later was known internationally for his feats of long-distance aviation. In 1932 he instituted the National Aviation Day displays. Using up to fourteen aircraft and a team of experienced flyers, he thrilled crowds with his daredevil stunts and also took paying customers for joy rides. It has been suggested that some of his aerial antics were performed at Low Hall and the photographic evidence appears to show that on occasions his aircraft were kept there. A nice little research project for an inquisitive mind would be to discover if Alan Cobham's aircraft were actually used in aerial displays at Low Hall or just parked there.

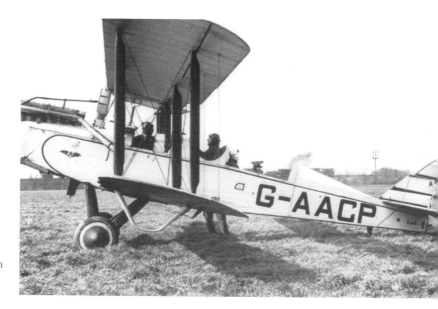

A two-seater de Havilland 9 biplane turned into a three-seater. Sitting in the centre, the pilot's position, is Sir Alan Cobham. The photograph was taken in April 1932.

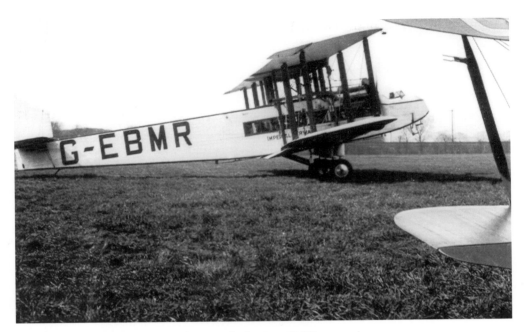

One of two Handley Page W10 biplanes, parked at Low Hall Farm, on loan to Sir Alan Cobham from Imperial Airways. These aircraft were each powered by two 450hp Lion engines.

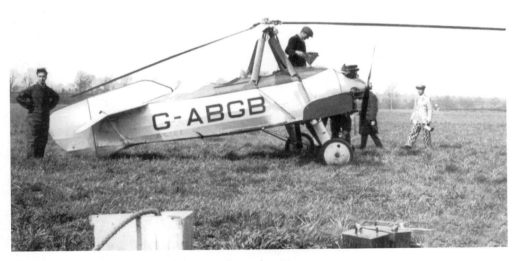

Refuelling an autogyro at Low Hall Farm ready to take visitors on a sightseeing trip to Wembley Stadium for the 1932 Cup Final. Alan Cobham charged his passengers £2 per head for the pleasure, a very reasonable amount compared to prices today.

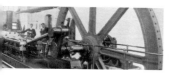

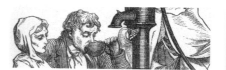

5. TOTTENHAM'S VICTORIAN LEGACY TO HEALTH

An early map of Tottenham showing Marke Fields (centre top), the source of the name Markfield.

Tottenham residents and visitors to the area who happen to enter the Broad Lane one-way traffic system at Tottenham Hale are probably unaware that between the River Lea and the railway, within a green space called Markfield Park, is a Victorian building that conceals a secret. However, residents of a certain age may find it easier to recall Tottenham Hale's vanished industries like Keith Blackman, Lebus and Gestetner that brought jobs and prosperity to the region. The products they made and the services they provided can be said to have helped shape our modern world.

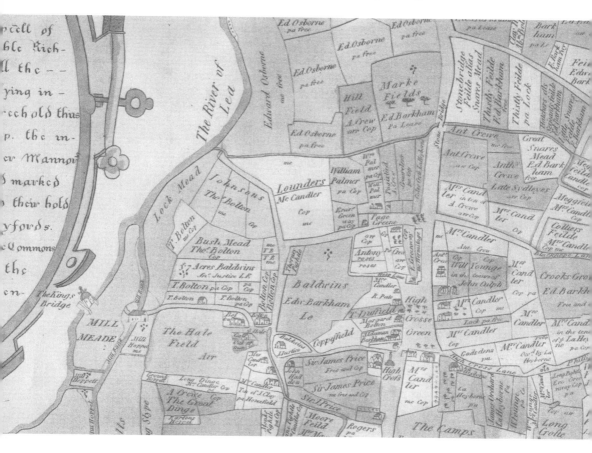

While it is easy to appreciate those structures in our community that provide our quality of life by producing goods and jobs, it is a simple matter to forget a crucial service, bequeathed to us by our Victorian ancestors, that continues to underpin the health and well being of everyone. The service referred to, sometimes considered too delicate to talk about in polite conversation, is the treatment and disposal of sewage. Perhaps, when we dutifully pull the chain or turn the handle to flush the toilet, it is a question of out of sight, out of mind. It is probably hard to imagine that in the early part of the nineteenth century, less than one hundred and seventy years ago, around the time when Queen Victoria came to the throne, infant mortality in British towns was bordering on fifty percent. Children were dying of conditions that are easily preventable today, such as typhoid, diarrhoea, dysentery and cholera. London, in the nineteenth century, was struck by epidemics of both cholera and typhoid that claimed the lives of thousands.

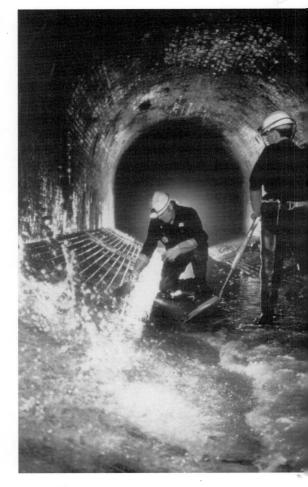

Thames Water workmen jetting a sewer to remove the build up of fat and other solids. The brick-lined tunnel is part of Bazalgette's Victorian London sewerage system that is still keeping the residents of the Metropolis healthy today.

While we are aware today of the importance of personal hygiene and the need to have clean drinking water, Victorian medical science had not generally progressed to this state of understanding. In 1844 a leading chemist, a Professor Booth, had considered that "free currents of air" circulating from the River Thames were the cause of London's ailing health. The eminent scientist, Michael Faraday, recognised the poor state of the Thames – he'd described it in a letter to *The Times*, July 1855, as a "fermenting sewer" – but seemed more concerned about the pungent smell than the possibility that it might be a source of disease. The concept of diseases being spread by air pollution, the "miasmic" theory, appears to have been a fairly common notion for many Victorians. It is claimed that even the famous "lady with the lamp", the nurse of the Crimea, Florence Nightingale, went to her grave in 1910 still believing in the theory.

Further evidence of the general acceptance of the miasmic theory amongst some of the most prominent men in the land can be gleaned from the reports of

An engraving 'Death's Dispensary' depicting how diseases like cholera could be spread by infected water. It was Dr John Snow (1813–1858) who first realised that the spread of cholera was due to sewage leaching into drinking water. In the cholera epidemic of 1854, Snow had the handle taken off a water pump near his Soho surgery and proved that his observations were correct.

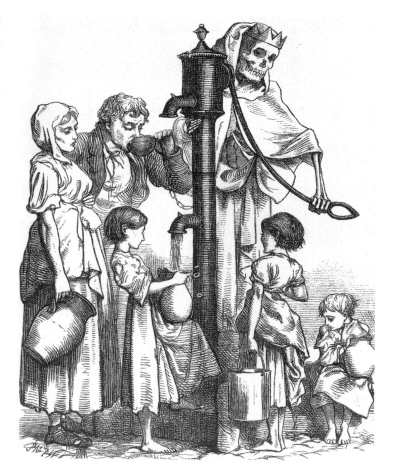

the "Great Stink" during the very hot summer of 1858. This was the year when the tidal flow of the Thames brought filthy effluent – discharged by citizens and local authorities alike into various water channels, and leached from overflowing cesspits into the river – as far up-river as the Houses of Parliament. In an effort to eliminate the dreadful smell, curtains soaked in chloride of lime were hung over windows and doors, presumably in the hope of protecting the members from the miasmic effect. It has also been reported that the then Chancellor of the Exchequer, Benjamin Disraeli, was seen leaving the House with a handkerchief clasped firmly to his nose. It was probably the Great Stink, more than anything else, that helped to cut through all the bureaucratic delays and financial hold-ups that Joseph Bazalgette, the Chief Engineer to the Metropolitan Board of Works, had endured. In the same year he was finally allowed to begin the task of building the London sewerage system. For its day the project was a truly massive civil engineering undertaking. Not only

were 1,300 miles of sewers to be completed including their main
northern and southern outfall pumping stations, but roads had to be
redesigned and aligned, bridges improved, and (a mammoth task)
embankments constructed on either side of the River Thames. The
design of the system was not just about handling the safe disposal
of London's sewage: it also had to cope with the drainage problem,
particularly in times of high rainfall.

Tottenham, by the middle of the nineteenth century, like other areas
of London, was suffering the effects of an expanding population,
which placed considerable pressure on the antiquated methods of
sewage disposal. By the late 1840s, it is estimated that around eight
hundred dwellings were discharging their effluent waste into the
Moselle Brook, which connected to the River Lea, itself a main
artery to the Thames. It would appear that the authorities had
identified the problems: in 1850, Tottenham became one the first
boroughs in Middlesex to take powers under the 1848 Public
Health Act to establish a permanent Local Board of Health. The
Board consisted of nine members who had financial powers
allowing them to put in place plans for a public water supply and
a system for the disposal of sewage.

A site adjacent to the River Lea, at the end of Markfield Road, was
chosen as the preferred spot for the sewerage works. To deal with
the effluent waste, a forty-five horsepower horizontal steam engine
was installed, driving a single double-acting pump. Incoming
sewage to the works was pumped to a pair of settlement and

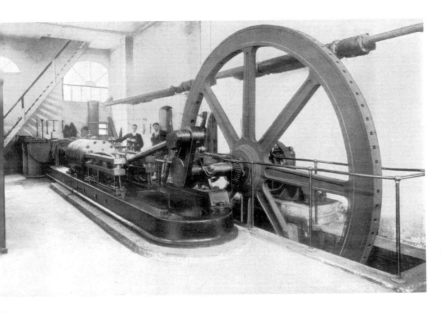

The first engine to be
installed at Markfield to
pump sewage sludge, a 45hp
horizontal condensing type.

holding tanks where the liquid effluent was passed through a series of sand filters and eventually discharged into the River Lea. Solids were removed from the site by a local manure contractor who had the responsibility for treatment before selling it on to neighbouring farmers. Two workmen lived on site in a pair of small purpose-built cottages. Their job was to provide twenty-four hour security, maintain the steam engine and stoke the boiler. By mid-nineteenth-century standards, it could be argued that Tottenham now had a relatively efficient sewage treatment and disposal system.

A sculpture of a river god, commissioned by the East London Water Works Company in 1809 for their original works at Old Ford. The sculptor was Joseph Theakston (1772–1842). After the site closed, the sculpture was taken to the Lea Bridge Water Works. When Lea Bridge closed, the River God was removed and given pride of place, in 1971, in front of Thames Water's Coppermill Lane site.

By 1853, the Local Board of Health claimed to have completed their arrangements to supply clean drinking water to all the built-up areas of Tottenham. However, by 1856, due to increased demand, it was found necessary to extend the water works at Tottenham Hale and water was abstracted from the surrounding marshlands. In 1858 a major problem occurred for the Board with the death of the local manure contractor. For some unaccountable reason, the sewage solids were not collected and the upshot was that the effluent was allowed to overspill onto the adjacent marshland and some was deliberately discharged into the River Lea. Eventually, the water that was being abstracted by the water works became contaminated due to the leaching of sewage through the soil.

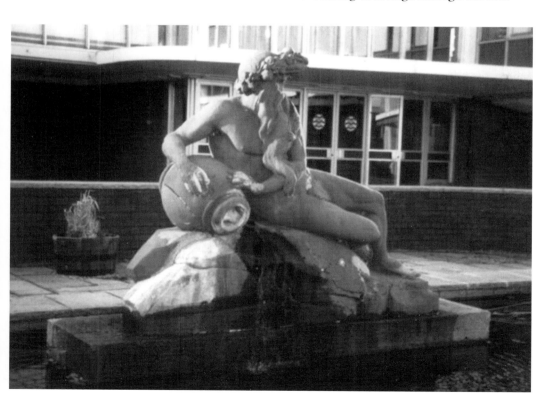

In 1866, a typhoid epidemic in east London caused the deaths of almost four-thousand people. The East London Water Works Company (ELWWC), established at Old Ford in 1807, had supplied many of these residents with water. The Metropolitan Water Act of 1852 had granted the company permission to build new reservoirs at Lea Bridge and also further north up the River Lea at Walthamstow. Because of Tottenham's effluent discharges into the river the ELWWC accused them of causing the deaths of their customers. While Tottenham's discharges were clearly not in the best interests of public health, the accusations, by the ELWWC, could have been a smoke screen to divert blame.

One of the provisions of the Metropolitan Water Act of 1852 was to ensure that reservoirs within a five-mile radius of St Paul's Cathedral should be covered. In September 1866, a group of twenty-nine residents (the Act provided for a minimum of twenty to complain) supplied with water by the ELWWC brought a complaint to the Board of Trade, claiming that the water supplied by the company was in fact contaminated water from the River Lea. A Captain Tyler was appointed to investigate the truth of the matter and found that on at least three occasions during 1866, the company was clearly in breach of the 1852 Act as water had been taken from an old uncovered reservoir, that was subject to contamination, and fed to one of their closed reservoirs, used for supplying drinking water. Tyler also concluded that between July and August 1866 an estimated 4,363 deaths had occurred, 3,797 of these being in areas supplied solely by the ELWWC. There were a further 264 deaths in an area shared with the New River Company, making the ELWWC wholly or partially responsible for over ninety percent of the fatalities.

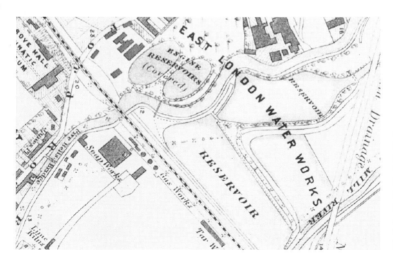

A detail from a map of 1862 showing two 'covered' reservoirs of the East London Water Works Company (ELWWC) at Old Ford. Covering was a requirement, under the Metropolitan Water Act of 1852, for reservoirs within a five-mile radius of St Paul's Cathedral.

As the nineteenth century progressed, the relocation of industries from east and central London to the relatively inexpensive Tottenham and other upper Lea Valley areas, brought increasing pressure on them to boost levels of sewage treatment and disposal, along with the supply of clean drinking water. The expansion of the Great Eastern Railway network into the region, with the offer of the cheap workman's ticket and the later introduction of the electric tram, made the area popular with commuters who were able to follow the jobs. It was not long before builders with an eye for business realised there was a growing market for affordable houses, further applying pressure on the Local Board of Health.

In 1885, things came to a head with the publication of a highly critical River Lea Conservancy report which stated, among other things, that "the real source of the condition of the Lea, other causes apart, was the neglect of the Tottenham Board… not providing sufficient tank accommodation for their rapidly expanding district". It would therefore appear that in a relatively short space of time, the once forward thinking local board had allowed the provision of public health to descend into chaos.

To address the problems, the Local Board consulted an experienced surveyor who came up with a seven-point plan to expand the Markfield sewerage works considerably. However, only two of the surveyor's recommendations were implemented, those of installing a new beam engine and increasing the length of the current settlement and holding tanks. By January 1886 the construction of a new engine house was completed and by November of that year Messrs Wood Brothers, of Sowerby Bridge, Yorkshire, had installed a hundred horsepower beam engine to drive two single-acting plunger pumps. The efficiency of the engine, commissioned on 12 July 1888, was such that over a twenty-four-hour period it could pump four million gallons of sewage sludge while turning at only sixteen revolutions per minute. Together with this new engine, powers granted under the 1886 Lee Purification Act and the construction of a new sewer linking into the Hackney Branch Sewer allowed the Markfield works to discharge the borough's effluent waste directly into Bazalgette's London sewerage system, for onward transmission to Beckton. Waste was no longer discharged into the River Lea as in the past. Not surprisingly, within a few years of these new arrangements the Lea Conservancy reported, "fish are now numerous in the river below the Tottenham Sewage Works".

By the early twentieth century, with a rapidly growing population, the issue of sewage disposal had to be readdressed yet again, thanks

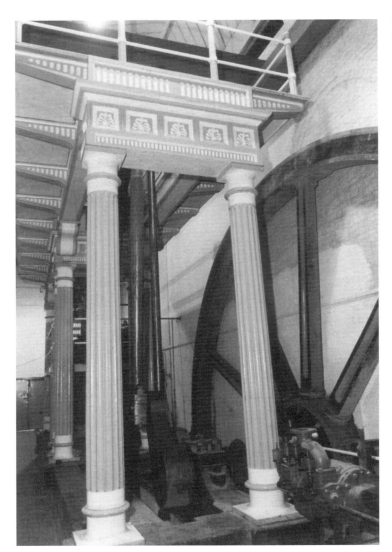

In 1886, a 100hp beam engine, built by Wood Brothers, Sowerby Bridge, Yorkshire, was installed at the Markfield site. It was the second engine to be installed at Markfield. The engine is the only example of its type that survives in the Lea Valley.

to the short sightedness of the Tottenham Local Board of Health and their failure to implement all the recommendations of their surveyor. In 1905, a second engine house had been completed by a local builder, Rowley Brothers of South Tottenham, in which three Worthington steam engines were installed along with six double-action plunger pumps and eighteen steam cylinders. The system was powered by any of three Lancashire boilers, two old and one new. The works' total pumping capacity increased by seventy-five percent to twenty million gallons in a twenty-four-hour period, allowing it to handle elevated levels of storm water. Under normal running conditions the plant would be limited to pumping ten

A picture of the Markfield engine taken in the early twentieth century with a workman proudly posing with an oil can in his right hand.

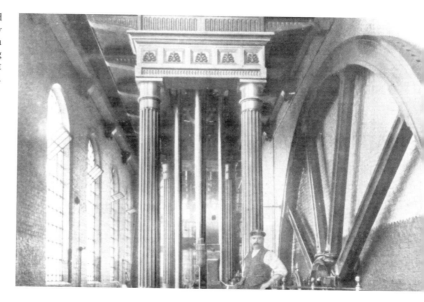

million gallons of sewage per day. Because of the increased pumping capacity of the works, an extra sewer had to be laid in parallel with the original. The total cost of all the building work and the installation of all the equipment came to £43,800.

Now that the installation of the new plant was complete, the forty-five horsepower pumping engine, installed in the early 1850s, was scrapped. The faithful Wood Brothers beam engine was retained, however, and remained on standby in its original engine house in case of emergencies. It was planned only to bring the engine online if storm water levels appeared to be rising at a dangerous rate.

A picture of the two engine houses at Markfield, probably taken in the early twentieth century.

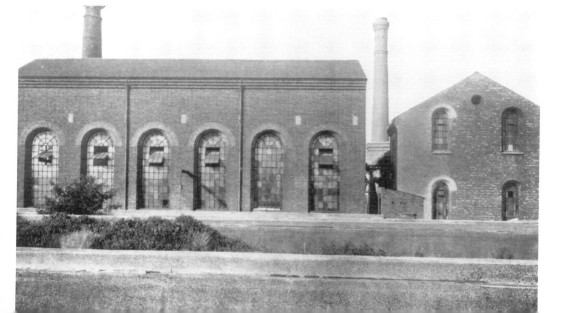

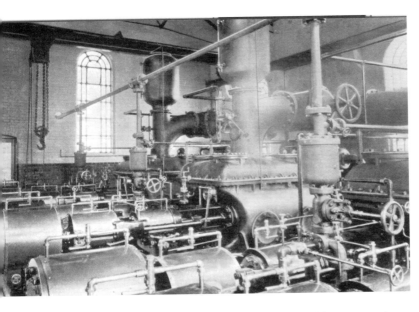

In 1905, three sets of triple-expansion horizontal Worthingtons, powered by Lancashire boilers, were installed at Markfield and the original 45hp engine was scrapped. A new engine house had to be built to accommodate the new plant.

The installation of the new facilities at Markfield seems to have been eminently timely. Only the year before, the furniture maker Harris Lebus (by the late 1940s, the largest in the world) opened a brand new factory on a thirteen-and-a-half acre green-field site at Tottenham Hale. As many employees had to travel to work from London's east end, Harris encouraged builders to create affordable homes for his workers locally, causing considerable expansion of South Tottenham's housing stock.

One of the three Lancashire boilers that supplied the Worthington engines with steam.

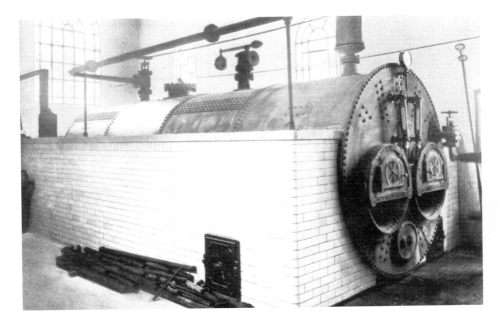

By the 1930s, because of the vast increase in the development of industrial, commercial and residential buildings across the region, Middlesex County Council had taken responsibility for the treatment of sewage. To address the problems that the increase in building had brought, plans were drawn up for the construction of a new sewage works to the west of the County at Mogden Lane, Isleworth and another in the east at Deephams, then in the borough of Edmonton (now Enfield). The Mogden Lane works were completed ahead of the Second World War, but Deephams' construction was postponed and not finished until 1963.

Like other areas of London, Tottenham suffered in the Second World War from the Luftwaffe's nightly raids. During the autumn of 1940, the engine house sustained damage in three of these, mainly to its roof, from incendiary and explosive devices. Fortunately, the Markfield engines were able to keep working for the duration of the War. During this period, alongside the essential sewage-treatment facilities, a pig farm with a house for the manager was built on the site as a way of boosting wartime food production. Local residents were encouraged to deposit waste food in bins specially provided at street corners. The contents of these were collected and processed by the local authority and turned into a source of animal feed that became affectionately known as "Tottenham Pudding". So it can be seen that the idea of recycling household waste is not a particularly new phenomenon.

Queen Elizabeth (the late Queen Mother) visiting the pig farm that was established at Markfield during the Second World War.

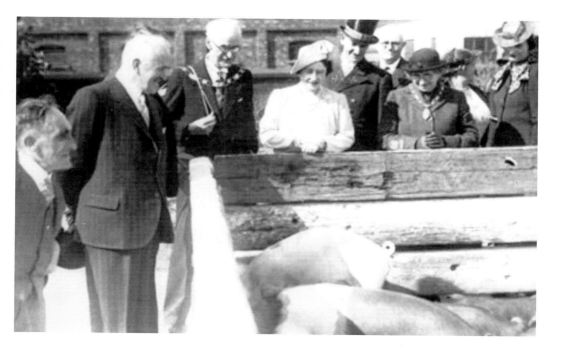

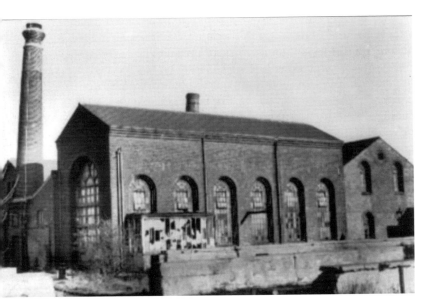

Markfield sewage pumping station was closed in 1965 and over the years became a target for vandals. The engine house windows were bricked up to protect the beam engine and in 1972 English Heritage conferred Grade II listing on the building.

The completion of the Deephams sewerage works in 1963 led the new London Borough of Haringey, now responsible for Markfield, to close the site and transfer its role to the new plant. A trunk sewer was dug from the Markfield works to the new facility, located in Edmonton only a few miles to the north, and was arranged so that sewage would flow under gravity. Now that Markfield's pumping provision was redundant, in February 1964 the works were finally closed and the surrounding site levelled. Over the coming years, as might be expected, the lonely buildings in their isolated location inevitably attracted the attention of vandals and the engine house sustained more damage from them than the Luftwaffe had ever inflicted. However, it was not until 1974 that the windows of the engine house were bricked up to protect the historic beam engine inside, and the site's accumulated rubbish removed.

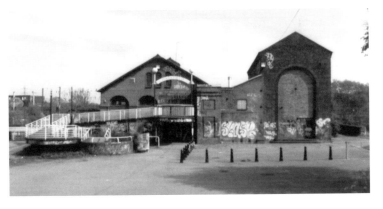

Markfield engine house today (2008), vandalised by graffiti artists.

The remains of the Markfield sewerage settlement tanks, heavily vandalised.

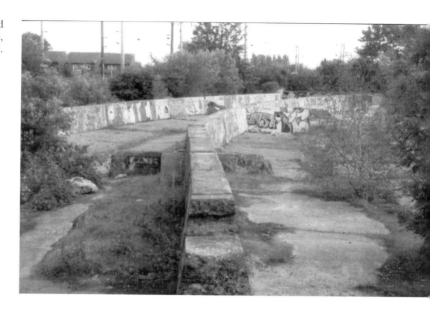

Luckily, a small group of enthusiastic volunteers recognised that something had to be done to protect this part of Tottenham's industrial heritage. They came together and formed what eventually became the Markfield Beam Engine and Museum Ltd., a company limited by guarantee and a registered charity, with the aim of maintaining and renovating the engine and also the building. This action has probably prevented the loss of what is believed to be the last engine manufactured by Wood Brothers. It is certainly the only surviving eight-column beam engine still residing in its original location.

The quality of the material used in the Wood Brothers engine can be gauged from the following single sentence written by G.R. Stephens, the Borough Engineer and Surveyor, in October 1984: "The Worthingtons finally succumbed to red rust (for the first time in their lives!!) and were scrapped". The Worthington engines were almost twenty years younger than the Wood Brothers' beam engine.

To help secure the future of the engine house, the Museum applied to English Heritage for listing and was eventually awarded Grade II status. The Museum's ultimate goal is now to make the beam engine a working exhibit, thereby creating an exciting visitor attraction. It is planned that visitors will be transported back into the past by the sight of the monster engine belching steam, the great horizontal beam rocking on its pivot point and the flywheel spinning. The Museum also wants to ensure that the site provides a first-class educational facility for young people, particularly groups from local schools who will be encouraged to become involved in simple research and other projects related to the site.

At the time of writing, in late 2008, the author learned that Markfield Beam Engine and Museum Ltd. had become the only project in London to qualify for a grant under the Heritage Lottery Fund's 'Parks for People' scheme. This has encouraged the local authority to get behind the Markfield project and assist the volunteers with their ultimate goal. The volunteers are also receiving considerable support from the curator and staff of Bruce Castle Museum and it is refreshing to see all these agencies working together. However, it is probably fair to conclude that if it were not for the vision and dedication of a small group of enthusiasts, an important part of our industrial heritage would have been lost to future generations forever.

REFERENCES

Author unknown, "The Opening of Outfall Works Extension", Tottenham and Wood Green Joint Drainage Committee, July 1905.

Author unknown, "Fit to Drink", Walthamstow Antiquarian Society, 1986.

Brereton, Kenneth, "The Site History of the Markfield Beam Engine", Markfield Beam Engine and Museum Ltd., 2007.

Clark, Dr Frederick, Secretary of the Markfield Beam Engine and Museum Ltd., personal conversation, August 2007.

Halliday, Stephen, *The Great Stink of London: Sir Joseph Bazalgette and the Cleansing of the Victorian Metropolis*, Sutton Publishing Ltd., Stroud, Gloucestershire, 2001.

Hedgecock, Deborah, Curator of Bruce Castle Museum Tottenham, personal conversation, August 2007.

Lewis, Jim, *London's Lea Valley: Britain's Best Kept Secret*, Phillimore & Co. Ltd., Chichester, 1999.

Lewis, Jim, *East Ham and West Ham Past*, Historical Publications, London, 2004.

Parliamentary Papers, 1867, Vol.58: "Report of Captain Tyler to the Board of Trade, in Regard to the East London Waterworks Company".

Note
The author has been informed by staff at Bruce Castle Museum that some pre-Second World War maps show a smallpox hospital located on the site of Markfield Park and it appears that little is known of its history. Also, by the same source, the author was informed that a local resident had recently reported that there was once an animal slaughter house on or near the site of Markfield Park and this has raised the question, did it have anything to do with the wartime pig farm? These are two more subjects that would make great research projects, as suggested above, for local schools.

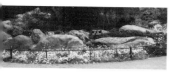

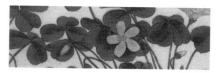

6. THE LEA VALLEY'S KEW GARDENS

The Lea Valley once had its own botanical gardens on a scale to rival those at Kew. Founded in 1759, the Royal Botanical Gardens at Kew in southwest London developed out of the plant collection of Princess Augusta, widow of Frederick, Prince of Wales and daughter-in-law of George II. Under the influence of the renowned botanist Sir Joseph Banks – who had accompanied Captain James Cook on his first voyage to the Pacific (1768–1771) – the gardens were increased in size and more exotic plants were acquired. In 1840, by now world famous, they were given to the state. The gardens once in the lower Lea Valley at West Ham, in contrast, were the result of the great passion for the study and collecting of plants of one private individual, Dr John Fothergill.

Despite being neither royal nor a great landowner, Fothergill's passion produced a botanical garden that Joseph Banks himself compared to the "royal munificence" of Kew. Born on 8 March 1712

In 1762, Dr John Fothergill purchased Upton House in West Ham along with about thirty acres of land. The house later became known as Ham House and was demolished in 1872. A stone kern, constructed with material said to have come from Ham House and Fothergill's rock garden, now stands in what is now West Ham Park close to the site of the original house.

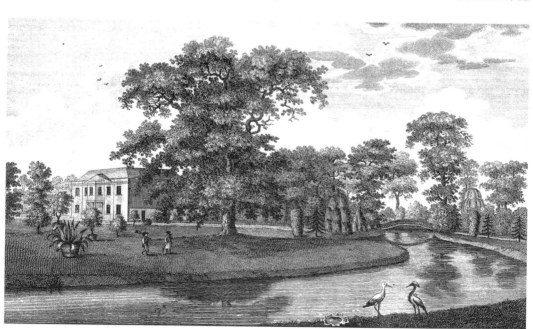

in a small stone farmhouse at Carr End, Wensleydale, Yorkshire, the second son of a Quaker, Fothergill was apprenticed to an apothecary in Bradford at the age of sixteen. In 1734, to further his chosen profession, he became a student at Edinburgh University and attracted the attention of the eminent professor of anatomy, Alexander Monro, who encouraged the young man to train as a physician. Forthergill took Monro's advice and, after graduating in August 1736, he spent a further two years at St Thomas's Hospital in London taking a course in medical practice under Sir Edward Wilmot. Interestingly, we learn from Fothergill's biographer that the journey from Edinburgh to London took between six to nine days and was made by sea.

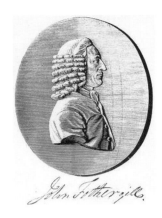

Dr John Fothergill (1712–1780) who was acknowledged for creating the finest private garden in Europe on the estate where he lived – now West Ham Park.

During his time of study at St Thomas's, Fothergill took it upon himself to read books on chemistry, botany and travel. In 1740, with his studies behind him, he made a short tour of Europe with a group of friends, returning in the same year to take up residence at 2 White Hart Court in the City of London where he set up as a physician.

During his training at St Thomas's Hospital, he had become acquainted with many poor people and it was they who sought him out when he set up in practice. To attend to the medical needs of these people, Fothergill often travelled across London, taking no fee for his services. While it is probably fair to say that he acted out of a genuine sense of kindness, and that these acts of charity were also a mark of his Quaker upbringing, it has been suggested by his biographer, R. Hingston Fox, M.D., that Fothergill gained considerable medical experience from these frequent acts of generosity. Fothergill's own view of the rewards of his charity is perhaps indicated by the remark, attributed to him, "I climbed on the backs of the poor to the pockets of the rich". This, in a way, allows us to understand something of the character of this remarkable man.

In 1744, Fothergill was admitted to the College of Physicians and by the age of thirty-six he had become one of the most respected practitioners in his field. Also, at about this time, he had established one of the largest practices in London. Fothergill took a great interest in, and made a study of, some of the more serious diseases that claimed the lives of Londoners, particularly those of children. This led him to conclude that the treatments of the day, normally bleeding and purging, were, in general, harmful to the patient. He therefore developed other less-intrusive regimes, in some of which he used a preparation of cinchona bark (from which we get quinine). These particular treatments were said to have had successful outcomes for his patients. In 1748, he published *An*

Account of the Sore Throat Attended with Ulcers. The book gained a wide readership and several editions were published, making him a much sought after consultant on this specialised subject. Further prestige was gained when, in 1754, he was elected fellow of his old college in Edinburgh and further honours came in 1763 and 1776 when he was elected both Fellow of the Royal Society in London, and Fellow of the Royal Society of Medicine in Paris.

In 1762, Fothergill purchased Upton House in West Ham along with about thirty acres of land, from an Admiral Elliot. Later, land adjacent to the estate was acquired and the gardens surrounding the house were enlarged. The grounds of Upton House became today's West Ham Park, which is one of the many open spaces, including Epping Forest, managed by the Corporation of London.

Shortly after he had moved to Upton House and only a little over two years after the foundation of the botanical gardens at Kew, Fothergill had begun to establish his own botanical gardens around his new home. It would appear that Fothergill did not just wish to develop his botanical gardens out of self-interest, nor purely as a means of collecting plants and shrubs for their intrinsic beauty and fragrance. He wished to introduce new species that might be used as the basis for new medicines and also for sources of food.

Fothergill introduced what was, for the day, leading-edge technology, building greenhouses and hothouses adjacent to Upton House. The largest of these was a hothouse measuring some 260 feet (80 metres) in length, in which he grew oranges and other tropical fruits. In all, some 3,400 different species of trees, plants and shrubs were collected and introduced into the gardens of Upton House. Fothergill's methods of enhancing his collection were quite imaginative. He approached ship's captains at the nearby London Docks and arranged with them to bring back barrels of earth and large interesting rocks as ballast from their overseas voyages. In many cases the barrels of earth also contained stowaways, in the form of seeds, which by accident had found the perfect way of being transported to Britain.

However, Fothergill did not rely solely on this method to procure his plants. He also corresponded with people throughout the world and obtained plants and seeds from places as far away as China and the West Indies. Collectors were employed to search the valleys and forests of North America while others were sent to West Africa. He had some scouring the Central European Alps in search of specimens for his newly created rock garden. It is claimed that the rock garden at Upton House was the first of its kind in Britain.

Sir Joseph Banks, by this time one of Britain's leading botanists, was so impressed with Fothergill's work that he decided to write, alluding to the great care and attention that had been give to the plant collection. In G. Thompson's *Memoirs of Fothergill*, Banks expressed the view that:

> At an expense seldom undertaken by an individual and with an ardour that was visible in the whole of his conduct, he procured from all parts of the world a great number of the rarest plants, and protected them in the amplest buildings which this or any other country has seen.

He also went on to write, with obvious enthusiasm, that the collection was:

> Equalled by nothing but royal munificence, bestowed upon the botanic gardens at Kew. In my opinion no other garden in Europe, royal or of a subject had nearly so many scarce and valuable plants.

Through his plant collecting, Fothergill had made many friends in America and, as a libertarian, had developed a great respect for the people of these British colonies. The mainly Quaker colonists of Pennsylvania were opposed, through their religious beliefs, to war and so were refusing to pay taxes, levied by Britain, for its prosecution. Along with other disputes over trade and taxes, this grew during the 1750s and 1770s and tensions between Britain and its American colonies were steadily mounting. In 1757, Benjamin Franklin, printer, author, diplomat, philosopher and scientist was sent to London by the Pennsylvanian Assembly to petition King George II over these matters. After carrying out his duties Franklin remained in Britain for five years, returning to America in 1762. In 1764, with tensions still running high between the two countries, Franklin again came to Britain as a representative of the Pennsylvanian Assembly. During the following eleven years of his residence in Britain, Franklin made many close friends. One of these was Dr Fothergill, who not only attended him as a physician but also became intimately involved in discussions with Franklin over the best possible ways of creating a breakthrough to reduce tensions and solve the political differences between the two countries.

In his later years, the demands on Fothergill as a physician and also his other work kept him away from his beloved botanical gardens. Management of the estate at Upton House was left to his fifteen gardeners. Occasionally, he would come by coach at night to visit the gardens and view his plants by lantern. Fothergill died in 1780

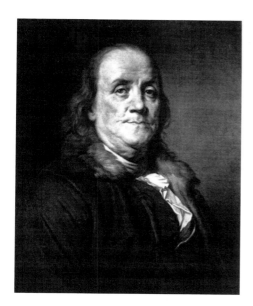

Benjamin Franklin
(1706–1790) printer, author,
diplomat, philosopher and
scientist.

and was buried at the Friends Burial Ground in
Winchmore Hill, north London. The headstone that
once marked his grave has been removed and the
caretaker in charge of the Burial Ground told the
author that it was taken to Ackworth School in
Yorkshire, an establishment that Fothergill had
founded.

Upton House was renamed Ham House and was
eventually acquired by the Gurney family, the well-
known philanthropic Quakers. In 1872, Ham House
was demolished and Fothergill's rock garden
removed. After a petition from the people of West
Ham to the Corporation of London to raise funds
for the preservation of the land as an open space,
sufficient capital was raised (with a generous
donation from the Gurneys) to open, in 1874, what
we now know as West Ham Park. A stone kern,
constructed with material said to be from Ham House and
Fothergill's rock garden, now stands in the park close to the site of
the original house. Fortunately, during Fothergill's lifetime he had
commissioned several famous artists to draw, paint and record his
plants, trees and shrubs. After Fothergill's death, Catherine the
Great, Empress of Russia, purchased approximately twelve hundred
of these pictures for £2,300, which, by today's standards, would
equate to several million pounds. Until recently, the pictures had
remained forgotten and unseen since their acquisition in 1781.

In the late 1980s however, the Chief Curator of the Komorov
Botanical Library in St Petersburg discovered a large quantity of

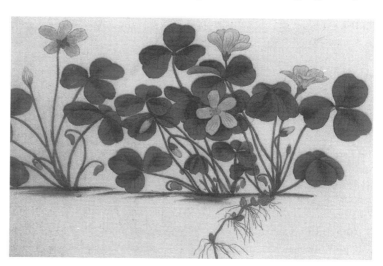

One of the pictures
commissioned by Fothergill,
discovered in the late 1980s
by the Chief Curator of the
Komorov Botanical Library in
St Petersburg.

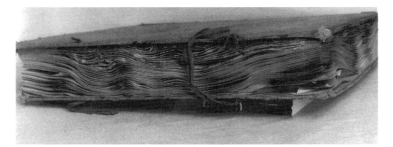

One of the original books of pictures discovered at the Komorov Botanical Library in St. Petersburg and waiting restoration.

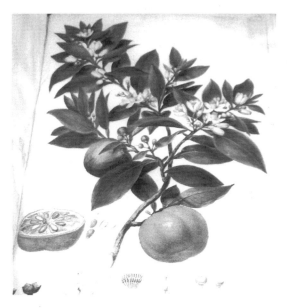

One of Fothergill's most famous artists, Georg Ehret, painted this picture, which is not among those that were discovered at the Komorov Botanical Library.

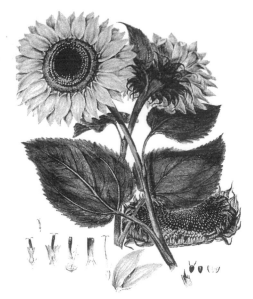

A picture of sunflowers commissioned by Fothergill and discovered at the Komorov Botanical Library. During his lifetime, Fothergill commissioned a number of artists to record his plant collection.

Fothergill's pictures still in their original wrapping. The author has been privileged to see a small selection of photographs that were taken of these pictures and has been genuinely astounded by their quality and exquisite colouring. Plans are currently in hand to bring the collection back to Britain so that delicate restoration work may be completed. The paper used for their production is in a poor state of preservation. Once restoration work has been completed it is hoped to put the collection on public display. This would provide a fitting memorial to Dr John Fothergill, a most remarkable man, who, through his love of plants, has been able to bring beauty into our lives long after his death.

The former Superintendent of West Ham Park, David Jones CBE, standing by the stone kern, which is said to have been erected close to the site of Upton House (later Ham House).

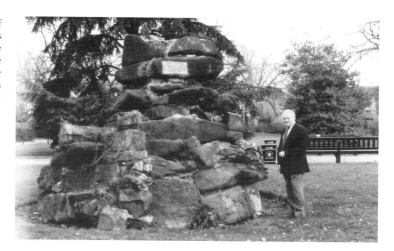

The author was extremely fortunate to be given a private tour of the gardens in West Ham Park by their most knowledgeable Superintendent, David Jones CBE, just before he retired from his position in 2002. Mr Jones pointed out a Maidenhair Tree (Ginko biloba) that had been planted in 1763, during Fothergill's time at Upton House. The tree had apparently flowered, for the first time, sixteen years after Fothergill's death when it was thirty-three feet (ten metres) tall. Mr Jones explained that the tree had been planted against the front wall of the former Upton House so that it could attract maximum sunshine and also warmth from the adjacent brickwork. A careful study of its trunk showed a flattened area that had presumably been shaped by the tree's close proximity to the building.

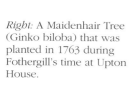

Right: A Maidenhair Tree (Ginko biloba) that was planted in 1763 during Fothergill's time at Upton House.

Far right: The trunk of the Ginko biloba tree showing a flattened area. This is thought to have been shaped by the tree's close proximity to Upton House.

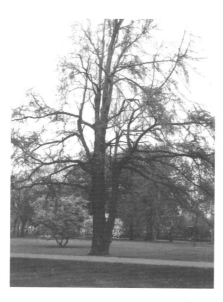

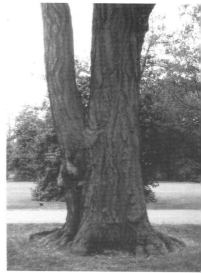

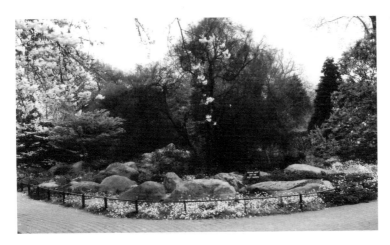

The rock garden in West Ham Park, imaginatively recreated by David Jones CBE in a style that Fothergill might have used.

During Mr Jones's time at West Ham Park he had carried out a programme of restoration and had also re-introduced a rock garden along with other plants and shrubs that had previously been grown by Fothergill. On the day of the author's visit (13 February 2002) a re-introduced tea tree plant had bloomed for the first time. This made the plant the first of its species to have bloomed in the gardens since Fothergill's day.

We should all be eternally grateful to those early pioneers like Dr John Fothergill who had the foresight, courage and determination to experiment with growing and cultivating unusual plants that were not native to this country. In this way, he has helped to increase our botanists and horticulturalists' understanding of ways that new plant species are propagated. In the longer term this has enabled growers to implement the cultivation of nutritious fruit and vegetables on a large scale. The benefits to health derived from such knowledge have proved a lifeline for millions of people around the world and the results are truly immeasurable, particularly if breakthroughs in the beneficial uses of certain plants as medicines are taken into account.

REFERENCES

Author Unknown, "Catherine the Great's lost Botanical Drawings", Cardington.

Fox, R. Hingston, *Dr. John Fothergill and his Friends*, Macmillan & Co. Limited, London, 1919.

Jones, David, Interview, February 2002.

Lee, Sidney (ed.), *Dictionary of National Biography*, Smith Elder & Co., 1909.

Lewis, Jim, *East Ham and West Ham Past*, Historical Publications Ltd., London, 2004.

Powell, W.R., *The Victoria History of the County of Essex*, Vol. VI, Oxford University Press, 1973.

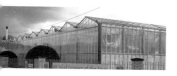
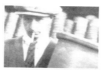
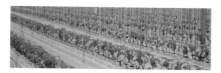

7. THE VALLEY THAT FED THE METROPOLIS

No book about the Lea Valley would be complete without mentioning the role of the glasshouse industry, which began to put down its roots (pardon the pun) in the upper part of the valley towards the end of the nineteenth century. Before this, there were several nurseries and market gardens in the lower part of the Lea Valley. Some of the earliest can be traced back to the seventeenth century, in areas such as Hackney, Clapton, Tottenham, Walthamstow and Edmonton.

The Lea Valley would seem to have been an ideal choice for those early growers wishing to establish their industry. Well-drained fertile loams and plentiful water supplies, from rivers and wells, were spread throughout the region. The navigable River Lea, linking directly to the River Thames and the capital's network of canals, could provide direct access for goods and produce to the markets of London. As the developing metropolis began its inevitable expansion in the Victorian and early Edwardian era, the lower part of the Lea Valley not only provided the space for the industrial move out of the capital, but also the much-needed land for workers' houses.

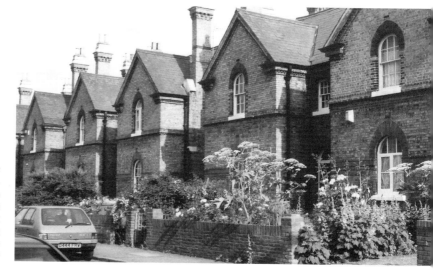

Some of the beautifully proportioned mid-nineteenth-century houses that were built in Abbey Lane for the workers and their families at the Abbey Mills Pumping Station. Will today's houses look this good 150 years on?

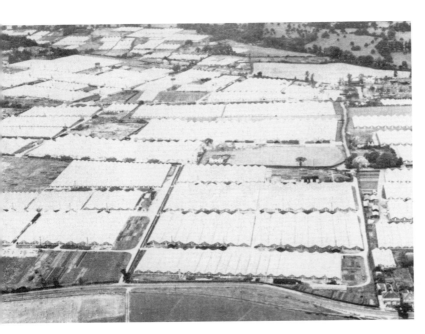

A view from the air, c.1960, of the concentration of glass houses at Cheshunt.

With the railway spreading its tracks northwards up the Lea Valley whilst industry and housing clamoured for space in the lower regions, the relatively undeveloped nursery land in the south became an obvious target for the developers. With the southern nursery land becoming a desirable commodity and the increasing amount of atmospheric pollution from the relocated factories, many growers came under pressure to move further northward up the valley to where the air was cleaner and the land cheaper. Gradually growers relocated their businesses and erected their glasshouses on open land in suburbs such as Enfield, Cheshunt, Nazeing and Waltham Abbey.

Peter Rooke, whose grandfather George set up in business as a Lea Valley nurseryman in the 1880s, suggests that the early-nineteenth-century nurseries "were little more than areas of ground where vegetables and garden bedding plants were grown in open air for the market". However, later in the century this changed with the development of the commercial greenhouse, encouraged, in 1845, by the removal of tax on sheet glass and improvements in heating and ventilation systems. By the 1930s, it is claimed, the Lea Valley had the world's largest concentration of greenhouses, with the Hertfordshire sector alone producing half of Britain's total horticultural output. This was now a major industry producing a wide variety of crops, with bulk supplies of tomatoes and cucumbers providing a cheap food source for the markets of Britain.

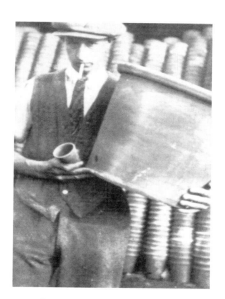

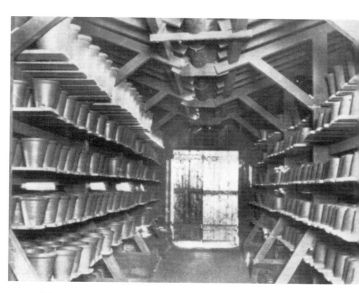

A workman with flower pots
of contrasting size at Messrs
South of White Hart Lane,
Tottenham, c.1927.

One of the flower-pot drying
sheds of Messrs South of White
Hart Lane, Tottenham, c.1927.

Many industries, particularly the motor manufacturers who
established themselves around Birmingham, encouraged providers
of parts and services to set up in business nearby to provide a
support infrastructure. The Lea Valley growers were no exception.
In Tottenham alone there were several manufacturers and
distributors of greenhouses, Duncan Tucker of Lawrence Road
being one of the largest. Samuel South and Sons, of White Hart Lane,
Tottenham, was a major supplier of a variety of clay flower pots to
the industry. This company manufactured its pots on site, having its
own clay pits, kilns and drying sheds.

By the start of the Great War (1914–1918) the Lea Valley growers
were developing into a major, and necessary, industry. In 1915, this
was recognised by government when, to support the growers, a
Research and Experimental Station was set up at Cheshunt by the
Ministry of Agriculture. However, in the years succeeding the
Second World War (1939–1945), the Lea Valley horticultural
industry began to come under increasing pressure from overseas –
as happened in manufacturing – from growers with the ability to
produce crops more cheaply. Initially, the Lea Valley growers
maintained an advantage over cheap imports into the UK, as the
cost of transporting this type of produce, which was essentially
perishable, was still prohibitive.

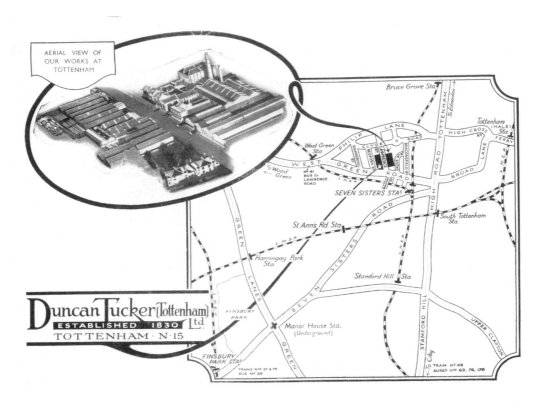

A view from the air, c.1936, of the Duncan Tucker factory at Lawrence Road, Tottenham (established 1830). Later, up until the 1980s, Thorn Lighting had a factory on this site.

With advances in technology, such as refrigerated vehicles and faster, larger aircraft, it became possible to have fruit and vegetables brought for sale in Britain from destinations never before considered a threat, often within twenty-four hours of harvesting. Many of these overseas growers, unlike their Lea Valley counterparts, were not constrained by the vagaries of the British climate which could saddle the UK grower with high heating bills. Even a switch from coal-fired heating to the cheaper and more efficient oil-fired systems in the 1950s could not prevent many growers from eventually leaving the industry. When this happened, the land on which the nurseries had stood was usually sold for building the swathe of new housing that, in many cases, would accommodate the workers who had moved out of London to follow their respective industries further up the valley.

Nowadays, the Lea Valley horticultural industry, which includes both edible and ornamental produce (flowers), is only approximately three hundred acres in area. In the 1950s, the figure was thirteen hundred acres. However, with the help of new technology and improved growing techniques, crop yields have increased dramatically – particularly those under glass. For example,

Her Majesty Queen Elizabeth the Queen Mother receives Mr and Mrs A.A. Pollard, being introduced by Mr L.C. Madsen. Following her Majesty is her brother the Hon. David Bowes-Lyon, Lord Lieutenant of Hertfordshire. The tour of the Lea Valley nurseries took place in 1959.

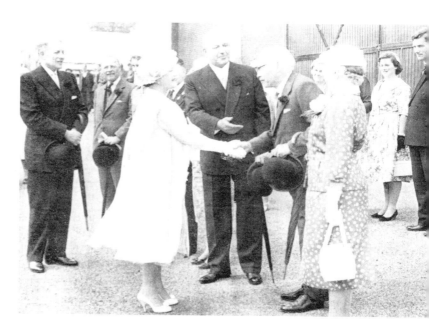

in the mid 1970s the yield for tomatoes was around seventy tons per acre; today the figure per acre is an astonishing two hundred and fifty tons. Cucumber production has also become more efficient with the Lea Valley growers producing one third of the nation's output.

Once, the Lea Valley's produce was directed towards the traditional markets of London, in particular Covent Garden and Spitalfields, with individual growers being responsible for grading, packing and transport. Now, due mainly to changes in the buying habits of the public, independent houses arrange the handling, grading and packing, with the support of computerised systems, before shipping the produce direct to the major supermarket chains. Often these retailers contract to purchase the entire output of a single grower. As it might be imagined, these new ways of working are achieved with a fraction of the labour force formerly employed.

General view of a block of cucumber houses, each 225 feet long by 15 feet wide, which once stood on a site near Waltham Cross, Hertfordshire.

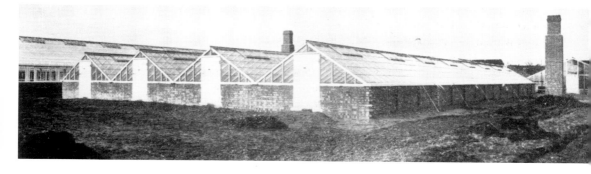

Major changes have also taken place within the house and bedding plant side of the industry, particularly in the areas of sales, marketing and production. The demise of internationally respected growers like Thomas Rochford at Turnford has left a gap in this sector of the market. With increasing public interest in gardening, brought about, in the main, by popular television programmes and magazines on the subject, the Lea Valley growers have yet again responded to the challenge. Concentrated in areas such as Crews Hill, Enfield and elsewhere in the valley there is now a substantial garden centre industry.

In localities like Crews Hill, relatively little growing takes place, although there is some preparation and production of bedding-plant packs for the increasingly popular superstore-type garden centres. The grouping of nurseries and garden centres in one place has resulted in a major attraction for the aspiring and serious gardener. Here the public are invited to buy not only plants direct from the suppliers, but also a staggering range of equipment. This includes garden ornaments, furniture, lighting, fencing, tools, sheds, paving, ponds and – not surprisingly – greenhouses.

While external pressures have brought many changes to the shape and structure of the Lea Valley glasshouse industry, the growers, supported by their own association, have always shown considerable resilience and ingenuity in the fight for survival. This has been particularly true in the face of cheap produce arriving from abroad from countries with lower labour costs and better climatic conditions than the UK.

A mark of the industry's resilience can be seen in the post-war period of the 1950s when it was difficult for the Lea Valley growers to attract and retain labour. Workers, at the time, were being enticed from horticulture to higher-paid jobs in the manufacturing industries located a short distance away down the Lea Valley. To counteract this trend, experienced workers were encouraged to come from Sicily and Italy to fill the vacancies. Several of these people worked extremely hard in the new country and in a relatively short time started businesses of their own, or took over existing nurseries.

The success of the immigrant community was such that, by the late 1970s, over fifty percent of the Lea Valley growers were Italian. With a further nine percent of businesses being run by people coming from other foreign countries, the British grower was now in the minority. However, it might be fair to speculate that without the intervention and support of the immigrant growers in the 1950s and 1960s, the Lea Valley glasshouse industry would not have developed into the competitive and efficient industry of today.

UPDATE

Since writing the above chapter a decade ago, a number of the Lea Valley growers have gone through another phase in their horticultural development. This has meant putting in high levels of investment, to keep the industry competitive in the face of stiff competition from abroad and the price demands of the large supermarkets.

VALLEY GROWN NURSERIES

One particular grower, Valley Grown Nurseries, has invested heavily in a series of hi-tech glasshouses using the CHP system (combined heat and power). Here, glasshouses with a floor space of six-or-more acres are growing peppers and aubergines (produce not seen before by the author in the region) along with the traditional crop of cucumbers. Gas has taken over as the preferred fuel from oil for heating the greenhouses, and the carbon dioxide (CO_2) produced in the process is fed into the growing areas and is naturally absorbed by the plants during the day, making a very efficient carbon-capture system.

Plants are now grown in individual containers and each is automatically fed a controlled amount of water and nutrients. The containers, which are filled with a rock-wool fibre mixture rather than earth or compost, are placed on what are termed "raised gutters". Effectively these are incredibly long shelves, suspended

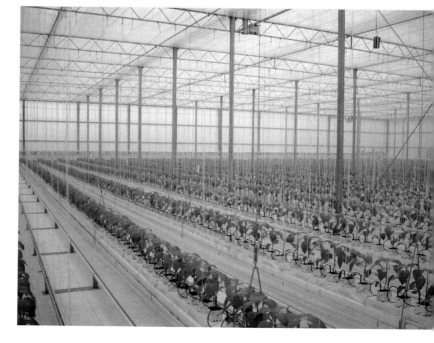

The scene from inside one of Valley Grown Nurseries' massive modern glasshouses showing thousands of pepper plants under cultivation. Note the system of "hanging gutters" now used by progressive growers in the propagation of plants.

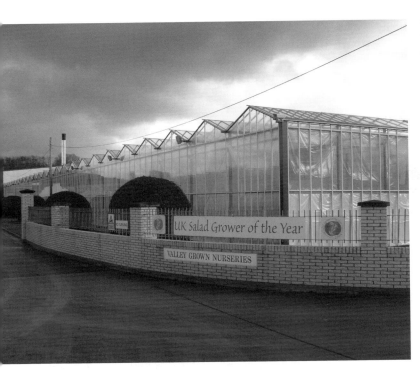

The entrance to Valley Grown Nurseries, which gives the visitor an immediate impression that they are entering a site of clean and efficient business.

above ground on a system of wire braces connected to the framework of the glasshouse. Thermal screens, which have around an eighty percent light transmission, are fitted approximately 3.5 metres above ground and 1.5 metres below the roof to reduce heat loss. The screens are computer controlled, as are most of the growing operations, pre-programmed by the grower to respond to the internal variations of temperature and light within the glasshouse. On entering these glasshouses the first impression one gets, apart from the vastness of scale, is the clean clinical conditions not too dissimilar from those to be found in a modern hospital.

GUY & WRIGHT LIMITED

Another Lea Valley grower, Guy & Wright Limited is a small third-generation family tomato-growing business in Hertfordshire, owned by John and Caroline Jones. The couple formed a partnership with Hennock Industries Ltd and New EnCo to develop a micro-turbine plant that would be powered from organic waste. To test the viability of the system, a working commercial plant was installed, partly funded by the Department of Trade and Industry (DTI) under the Technology Programme. After successful trials, the plant was enlarged and John and Caroline took the bold decision to move away from fossil fuels as the main power source, using them only as an alternative when the economics dictated.

THE ANAEROBIC DIGESTER CYCLE AT GUY & WRIGHT

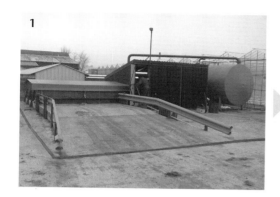

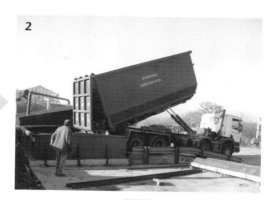

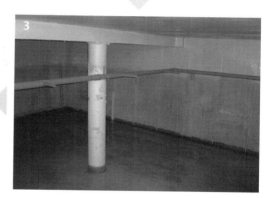

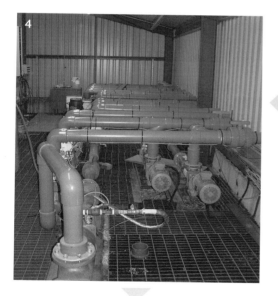

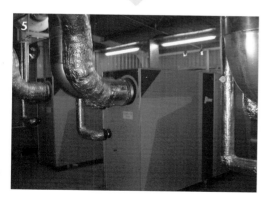

1   Organic waste reception area at Guy & Wright.

2   A delivery of organic waste to Guy & Wright that will be fed into an underground storage area before being reduced to a 'vegetable soup' by machinery.

3   An internal view of part of one of the six underground cells for holding vast quantities of decomposing organic waste. This material will eventually produce methane gas, through the anaerobic digestion process. The methane will drive micro turbines and electricity will be produced.

4   Picture showing part of the plant that is necessary to run the anaerobic digestion process for turning organic waste into gas, electricity and clean CO_2.

5   The gas-powered turbines that produce electricity to run the Guy & Wright Nursery. Surplus energy is sold to a green energy company to power people's homes.

To expand the system (known as anaerobic or oxygen-free digestion – see the next chapter for an explanation of how a typical system works), an enormous below-ground six-cell airtight bunker was constructed. Each cell is capable of holding four hundred tonnes of organic waste which, as it decomposes, produces biogas with a high methane content. The gas can be compressed to drive micro-turbines directly, a system of electricity production more efficient and cleaner than the traditional method: this required the burning of natural or town gas to heat water so that the resulting steam would drive turbines coupled to electricity generators. With the new system, the gas-burning stage of the process is completely eliminated.

The anaerobic digester in use by Guy & Wright is an exceedingly greedy animal, requiring fifty tonnes of organic material per day to satisfy its hunger. It would be impossible for the nursery to generate such a large daily amount of organic waste from its own operation, so arrangements have been made with London's Spitalfields Market, Bedfordshire Growers (who pre-pack onions), and the banana-importers J.P. Fresh of Dartford. These companies, and others, are all extremely grateful to donate their organic waste to Guy & Wright rather than send it to landfill which would incur them paying a levy. As an environmental initiative, it is an all-round win-win situation.

Waste material coming to the nurseries is emptied by the delivery vehicles into a receiving pit, from where it moves slowly to a macerator which crushes and breaks it down into smaller pieces. The resultant 'vegetable soup' is pumped into a holding tank before being distributed to the six underground digesting cells. This process is closely controlled by computer probes and only after testing and analysis does the required amount of material get fed to each of the cells. Waste residue from the cells is fed to three established reed beds, allowing the system to continuously supply gas without the need to shut down for cleaning. The biogas generated by the plant is fed into a giant inflatable bag which can then supply the five micro-turbines that produce the electricity and also a small boiler which is used to power the three miles of underground heating below the digestion cells. Being mainly devoid of sulphur, the CO_2 produced by the process is so clean that it can be fed directly, without any form of treatment, into the glasshouse growing area to be absorbed by the plants during the day. This arrangement has considerably improved crop yield.

The installation of the plant began in 2003 and took three years to complete, with much of the construction work done by the Joneses and local specialist contractors. As is to be expected with a plant so unique, initial teething problems occurred that had to be resolved alongside the Jones family running their business. With some understatement, Caroline Jones concedes that the plant installation "has been by no means easy" but now – and, I suspect, with some relief – she's able to say "we have achieved our goal".

Dr Andy Marchant of Hennock International Limited, the designer of the anaerobic digestion system at the nursery, has claimed that "John and Caroline Jones were the first growers in the world to install micro-turbines with high-rate CO_2 enrichment on a commercial nursery, and have been host to countless other growers keen to see what they were doing".

When the plant became fully operational the system produced more than enough electricity to satisfy the running of the nursery and the excess power was sold to Green Energy, a company that was established specifically to obtain and distribute electricity from renewable sources. This arrangement allows the Joneses to forget about the need for customer administration, with its inherent problems of metering and billing and to get on with the daily task of running their business.

For all their hard work, considerable financial expenditure and futuristic risk-taking, John and Caroline Jones rightly deserved the prestigious Grower of the Year Awards 2009 Business Initiative of the Year commendation.

There has been a decline in the number of Lea Valley horticultural growers over the past decade and the Joneses are the last remaining tomato growers in Hertfordshire; but overall the other specialists are still supplying the UK markets with a third of their cucumber requirements. Also, it should be remembered that in the 1970s the yield for tomatoes grown in the region was approximately 70 tons per acre. Now, with the new technology, it is typically 280 tons, with more varieties grown to satisfy changing consumer demands.

While it is not possible to predict the state of the Lea Valley horticultural industry over the next ten years, particularly in the current unprecedented harsh economic climate, those remaining growers who have made the commitment to provide us with salads produced in the most environmentally friendly way deserve the support of all the retailers and also us, the consumers.

REFERENCES

Author unknown, "Golden Jubilee of the Lea Valley Growers' Association – October 1911–October 1961", National Farmers Union, Hertfordshire, 1961.

Author unknown, "Collaborative Research and Development: Waste Minimisation", DTI Document, 2003.

Author unknown, "Retailers must take lead in fair pricing", *Lea Valley Growers' Association's Newsletter*, Issue 395, December, 2008.

Currie, C.R.J. (ed.), *The Victoria History of the County of Middlesex, Vol. X – Hackney*, University of London Press, London, 1995.

Franklin, Andrew, Valley Grown Nurseries, private conversation, January 2009.

Jones, Caroline, Guy & Wright Limited, private conversation and correspondence, January 2009.

Marchant, Dr Andy, "Grower of the Year Awards – Guy & Wright Ltd".

Rooke, Peter, "The Lea Valley Nursery Industry", *Hertfordshire's Past*, No. 42, Hertfordshire Archaeological Council, Hertfordshire, Autumn 1997.

Shaddick, Claire, "Grower Power", *The Commercial Greenhouse Grower*, May 2003.

Stevenson, R.A. (Tony), Lea Valley Growers' Association, private conversation and correspondence, June/July 1998 and January 2009.

Taylor, Gary, Valley Grown Nurseries, private conversation, January 2009.

Ward, Frank, Director, Hennock International Ltd, Nettleham, Lincolnshire, private conversation, January 2009.

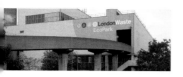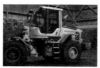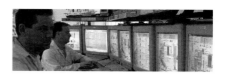

8. WHAT A LOAD OF RUBBISH!

Public health is intrinsically linked to environmental issues: no book that tried to tell its story would be complete without addressing the problems that all of us continue to create for our planet through the continuing generation, transportation, and disposal of household and industrial waste. Every year, in Britain alone, hundreds of millions of tonnes of waste are produced with large quantities of unprocessed material ending up in landfill sites, piling up environmental problems for the future. As we start our journey into the twenty-first century, nations around the world are beginning to wake up to the increasing dangers created by the melting of Arctic and Antarctic ice sheets, rising sea levels and severe droughts. These are some of the effects of global warming, caused by increasing emissions of methane (some from landfill sites), carbon dioxide and other polluting gasses such as CFCs (chlorofluorocarbons) that are destroying the protective ozone layer that surrounds our planet.

While the links between public health and waste disposal might not be immediately obvious, it is worth remembering that decaying and festering matter attracts vermin and can also lead to the spread of diseases. So it is important that our waste is disposed of in a controlled and efficient way that is sympathetic to the environment. This means recycling, rather than destroying, our precious materials and also making sure that toxic waste is not allowed to enter the food chain.

Humankind has been increasing pollution levels since time immemorial, but the process speeded up considerably during the Industrial Revolution in the eighteenth century. The burning of large quantities of fossil fuels, particularly coal, to power our factories – and the use of coal in the production of town gas, to light and warm our homes – has allowed the release of millions of tonnes of stored carbon dioxide. This harmful gas was trapped in the fossil materials for millions of years until our avaricious quest for more and more energy secured its release into the atmosphere.

Over the last two centuries there has been a rapid increase in deforestation in countries around the world, to provide both timber and land for farming, in particular large-scale agricultural schemes like the cultivation of soya and other crops in an effort to sustain a growing population. These large-scale programmes have contributed vastly to raise carbon emissions as the trees that capture carbon dioxide and give off life supporting oxygen are felled. The destruction of the trees has also caused soil erosion on a massive scale, which provokes landslides as dead roots can no longer provide a grip on the surrounding earth.

With the progress of time, improvements in technology have allowed us to harness the energy contained in other fossil fuels, such as natural gas and oil. From the refining of oil, a carbon-emitting industry in its own right, we obtain petroleum, plastics and a whole range of chemicals and fertilizers – and also the energy to drive power stations and other industrial processes. Natural gas is used by most of us to cook and heat our homes; but it also has many different uses for manufacturing everyday products that we have come to rely on, and so our industrial base would collapse without it. It is now a fact of life that fossil fuels have become a cornerstone of our way of life and our future survival. Unfortunately for us, they will not last for ever. In Britain, stocks of North Sea oil are dwindling and most of our coal mines have closed (some on economic grounds and not always due to the depletion of coal). So what is the solution to this dilemma? In short, being more careful in the use of our precious resources and dramatically changing our throw-away culture, into one of conservation and the recycling of all recoverable materials and waste.

For a number of years, north London has been at the forefront of an innovative scheme to turn apparently useless rubbish into a range of useful materials and also energy sources, like gas and electricity. The project referred to was first commissioned in 1970 by the former Greater London Council (GLC) and built on land adjacent to the Eley Industrial Estate, where the North Circular Road (A406) crosses the Lee Navigation. At the time of the project's conception it was known as the Edmonton Incinerator, and largely dealt with burning household and other waste to produce electricity. After much scientific research and planning, this original scheme has evolved into LondonWaste's EcoPark. This considerably improved facility, with its team of passionate and dedicated staff, has totally transformed waste handling and recovery into something that would have been unimaginable only a few years ago. However, as the author learned on a recent tour of the site, no member of staff is complacent or resting on their well-earned

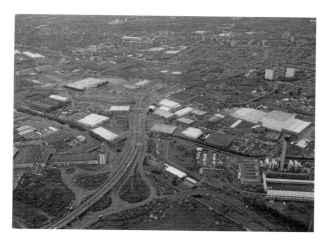

An aerial view of the North Circular Road (A406) looking west. To the right of the picture, where the road crosses the Lee Navigation, is LondonWaste's EcoPark, identified by the tall chimney.

laurels: there is an ongoing review and monitoring of their systems, research and techniques to find new and improved ways of waste recovery. The ongoing aim is to reduce the reliance on landfill sites and also to help the world's carbon footprint become smaller.

The simplest way to describe the operation of LondonWaste's Lea Valley EcoPark is to break it down into its dedicated recycling and recovery areas.

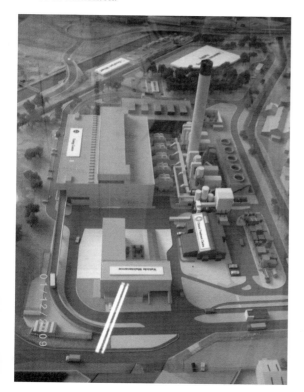

A model showing LondonWaste's main buildings, on display in the reception area of the Energy Centre at Edmonton.

BULK RECYCLING CENTRE

This is where the recovery and separation of materials takes place. After separation, the materials such as plastic, wood, fluorescent tubes, rubble, refrigerators and television receivers are stored. In order to keep to a minimum the journeys to and from specialist contractors, the separated materials are allowed pile up until they reach a required tonnage. In turn, the contractors then strip and process the various materials which will eventually be turned into new products.

COMPOST CENTRE

Green garden and kitchen-scrap waste arrives at the centre and a mechanical shovel deposits the material into the hopper of a large shredding machine. Once shredded, the material is transferred by conveyor where water sprays dampen it before it is deposited onto a great heap within the centre. After standing for

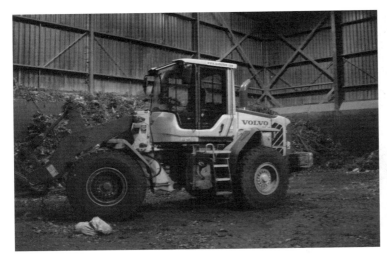

A mechanical shovel within the Compost Centre, used for arranging the biodegradable material within the building and also for placing it into the hopper of a large shredder. This machine reduces the bigger pieces of organic material, like discarded Christmas trees and so on, into more manageable chippings for the next stage of the composting process.

approximately twenty-four hours, the material is transferred into specially designed tunnels, each around thirty metres long. Here it stays for between two to three weeks as it undergoes the decomposition process, having controlled amounts of air forced through it. In the tunnels each batch of material will heat up to the required temperature of 60°C which must be maintained for two consecutive days to meet government guidelines. The process, which effectively takes place in a container, is called "in vessel composting". While the material is in the container the temperature, moisture and air flow are carefully monitored. This is done from a control room that takes regular readings from temperature probes located inside the tunnels.

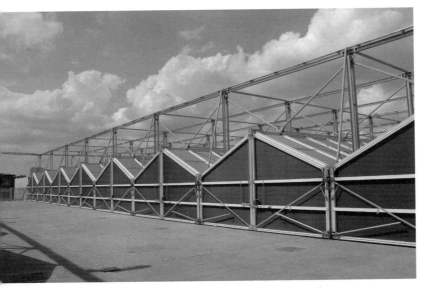

Material is taken from the Compost Centre reception building and placed in large thirty-metre-long containment tunnels where it will decompose. Here it stays for two to three weeks, decomposing and having controlled amounts of air forced through it.

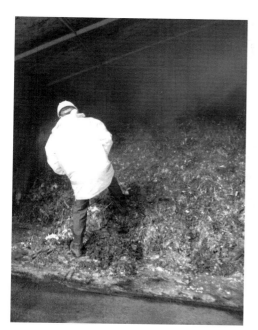

A workman examines the decomposing organic waste within a containment tunnel.

After a period of two to three weeks, the partially decayed material, by now odourless, is removed and placed in another series of tunnels and the whole process is repeated. This ensures complete breakdown of the waste. After remaining in the tunnels for the required time, the material is removed to an outside bay where it is allowed to cool to around 40°C during the maturing process. This can last up to ten weeks. The last process is screening where pieces of wood, plastic, stone and anything else considered too large are removed by sieves. Remarkably, the Compost Centre is capable of handling up to forty-five thousand tonnes of green garden and kitchen waste a year.

The quality of the compost produced is such that it meets the British Standards Institution's specifications and is used by a range of different agencies, including farmers, landscapers and local authorities. As might be imagined, the Compost Centre and LondonWaste as a whole are required to meet strict inspection standards imposed by the Environment Agency, the Health and Safety Executive and the State Veterinary Service. So confident are the management of LondonWaste regarding the maintenance of these particular standards that it has, of its own volition, given the inspectorate security access passes to the site allowing them to arrive unannounced at any time of day or night.

A view of LondonWaste's main building, the Energy Centre, at the Edmonton EcoPark, north London. The building houses waste processing and the boilers, turbines and electricity generators. Note the raised roadway to the right which allows the waste delivery trucks to enter and leave the building.

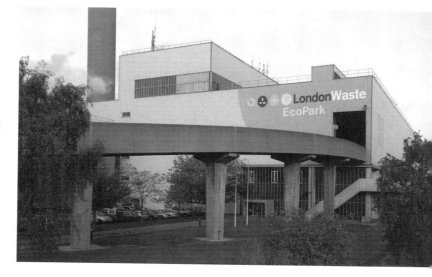

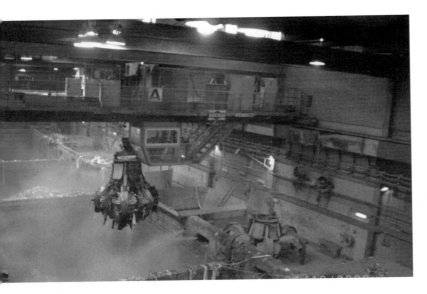

A mobile crane, with grab, loading mixed waste, unsuitable for recycling, into the feed hoppers of the main boilers. This type of waste would have otherwise gone to a landfill site. The heat generated, by burning the waste, turns water into steam to drive turbines. These, in turn, are coupled to the electricity generators and provide power to run the site. The surplus energy created is sold to the National Grid and provides power for around 56,000 homes. Note the mist above the waste hoppers: this is a fine water spray designed to keep dust levels in the plant to a minimum.

ENERGY CENTRE

When all the recoverable waste has been separated for processing, the left-over mixed material that would normally go to a landfill site is fed into massive furnaces, where combustion takes place at a minimum temperature of 850°C (although temperatures are usually maintained somewhere between 900°C and 1000°C). The heat generated by the furnaces is used to turn water into steam, which drives turbines coupled to generators that produce electricity. During a typical year, enough electricity is generated to keep the whole site self sufficient whilst the surplus, sufficient to power 56,000 homes, is fed to the National Grid. Flue gasses from the boiler chimney are scrubbed and passed through carbon and lime

The Turbine Hall, located within the Energy Centre at LondonWaste. This is where electricity is generated from the combustion of mixed waste that is currently unsuitable for recycling.

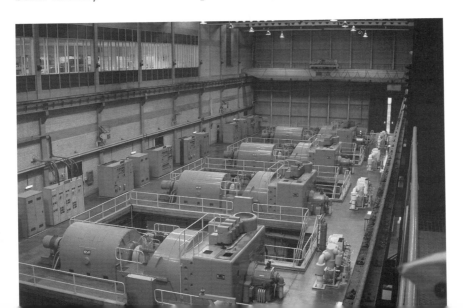

The control room, hub of the LondonWaste's Energy Centre operations. Here operators can monitor and control, from computer screens, all the functions in the waste recycling process from furnace temperatures to chimney emissions.

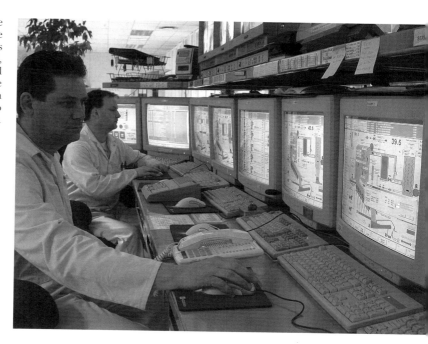

filters and are also subjected to Electrostatic Precipitators to remove harmful particles. Recently, an improved type of lime was introduced into the cleaning process, which has reduced considerably the need to mine large quantities of natural limestone. Materials that are known to produce high amounts of toxins are removed from the waste mix before they can be burned and the emissions from the chimney are strictly monitored by computers in the control room, ensuring the air quality around the plant remains clean.

CLINICAL TREATMENT CENTRE

The Clinical Treatment Centre is run by a wholly owned subsidiary of LondonWaste Limited, known as Polkacrest. It provides a safe and efficient clinical waste collection and treatment service for NHS trusts, private hospitals, nursing homes, dentists, doctors' surgeries and even tattoo artists. Perhaps some readers might remember the large factory-type chimneys that discharged liberal quantities of smoke and soot, by-products of the burning of clinical waste with coke (a combustible bi-product of the manufacture of town gas from coal). These chimneys graced the skyline behind many a Victorian hospital building and were accepted as part of the operation of the site.

Now that we know a little more about the harmful effects of pollutant discharges into the atmosphere, we should feel reassured by this replacement of an unhygienic and haphazard method with a modern efficient system of clinical waste treatment and disposal, contained within a specialist handling unit. Clinical waste is combusted at high temperature in a furnace and the resultant heat is used to produce steam to generate electricity. The process is similar to the way electricity is generated in the Energy Centre, mentioned above.

To ensure safe disposal and compliance with current legislation, LondonWaste operates a certification scheme for its customers. The certification scheme also applies to their sensitive-document destruction service.

ASH RECYCLING CENTRE

After the mixed waste material has been subjected to high temperature combustion in the furnaces to produce electricity, the remaining ash is examined by a specialist team of operators who remove any residual metals before it is recycled and graded. The end product is used as a secondary aggregate by the construction industry and therefore reduces the need to remove large quantities of natural materials from the earth.

WOOD CHIPPING CENTRE

Large quantities of wood, particularly old discarded pallets, are shredded into chips which can then be used for weed suppression around shrubs, covering for garden paths, animal bedding, fuel and also new wood-based products. Perhaps the person fly-tipping wood from a building site will end up purchasing quantities of particle board manufactured from the very waste he illegally dumped!

ECOPARK WHARF

LondonWaste is ideally situated adjacent to the Lee Navigation and has its own wharf. It is the vision of the company to take waste management to the next stage and it is actively exploring environmentally friendly ways of using the canal system to move waste in bulk to and from the site. If this could be achieved, with the help of government agencies, it would reduce considerably the need for large-scale road transport movements, reducing congestion and further helping to improve our environment.

FUTURE POSSIBILITIES – AN ANAEROBIC DIGESTION PLANT?

The recycling of waste materials is always under scrutiny and responsible companies are constantly on the lookout for new technologies that will improve current efficiencies. One such technology, anaerobic digestion (AD), involves processing biodegradable waste in an enclosed reactor vessel, effectively a large tank devoid of air. As the waste breaks down, a biogas is produced. This is largely made up of a mixture of hydrogen, methane and carbon dioxide. The process also produces sludge, which, after processing in the open air, can be spread on land as a fertiliser. To maintain the AD process, the reaction vessel has to be heated. After initial priming has taken place, the biogas created by the process is used to continue the heating of the waste, and any surplus gas is used for the production of electricity.

Anaerobic digestion is a tried-and-tested technology and is becoming increasingly popular around the world with a number of industries, especially agriculture, horticulture and farming. Nevertheless, it could prove costly to integrate such a process into the recycling of household waste. The biodegradable waste used is usually made up of vegetable and other food products. Therefore, it would be necessary to explore the economic logistics of storing; collecting and delivering the material to LondonWaste from households within the seven North London local authorities (Barnet, Camden, Enfield, Hackney, Haringey, Islington and Waltham Forest) that currently make up the main waste catchment area. Otherwise, the cost to local ratepayers might prove unacceptable.

IN CONCLUSION

The Lea Valley is fortunate to have the largest waste recycling and composting park of its type in Britain, dealing with our daily creation of rubbish in some of the most environmentally friendly ways yet devised. This is helping to lower the earth's carbon footprint by reclaiming useful materials that would otherwise go to landfill. Perhaps the northern saying "where there's muck there's brass" applies also in the south!

REFERENCES

Author unknown, "Recycling North London's Waste", LondonWaste Ltd, Edmonton.

Lord, W., "EcoPark – Treating Rubbish as a Resource", LondonWaste Ltd, Edmonton.

Scott, Nicky, *Composting – an Easy Household Guide*, Green Books, Totnes, Devon, 2005–6.

Staff interviews, LondonWaste Ltd, January 2009.

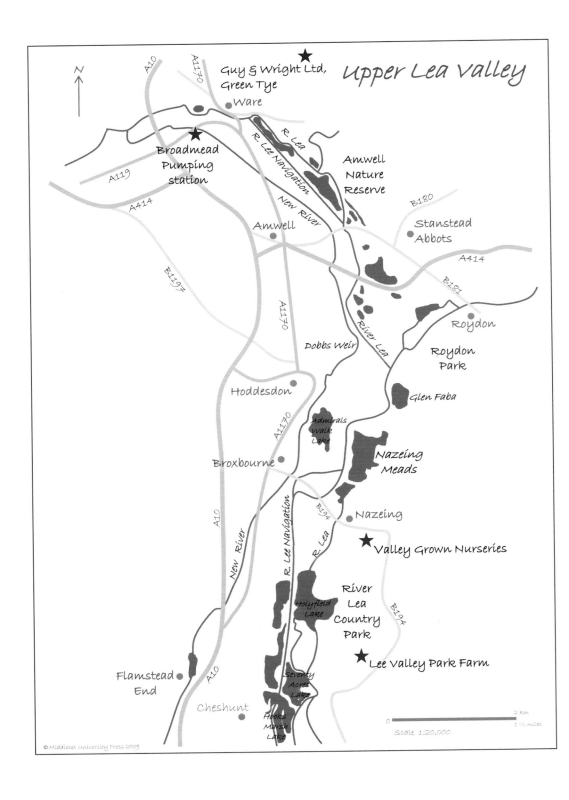

Upper Lea Valley

N

A10
A1170
★ Guy & Wright Ltd, Green Tye
● Ware
R. Lea
R. Lee Navigation
★ Broadmead Pumping station
A119
A414
New River
Amwell Nature Reserve
B180
Stanstead Abbots
● Amwell
A414
B1197
B181
A1170
Roydon ●
River Lea
Dobbs Weir
Roydon Park
● Hoddesdon
Glen Faba
A1170
Admirals Walk Lake
Nazeing Meads
● Broxbourne
A10
New River
R. Lee Navigation
B194
R. Lea
● Nazeing
★ Valley Grown Nurseries
Holyfield Lake
River Lea Country Park
B194
● Flamstead End
A10
Seventy Acres Lake
★ Lee Valley Park Farm
● Cheshunt
Hooks Marsh Lake

0   2 km
                1 ¼ miles
Scale 1:20,000

© Middlesex University Press 2009

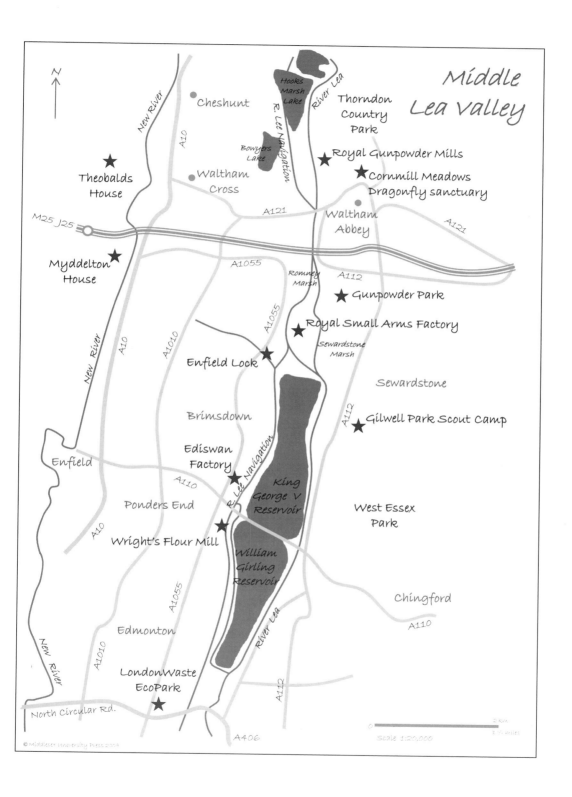

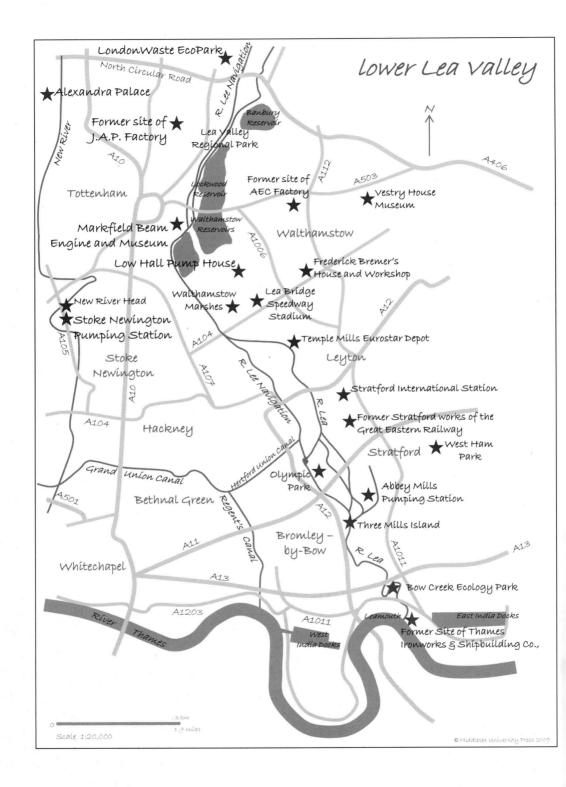

Lower Lea Valley

LondonWaste EcoPark

North Circular Road

R. Lee Navigation

Alexandra Palace

Former site of J.A.P. Factory

Banbury Reservoir

Lea Valley Regional Park

New River

A10

A406

A112

A503

Tottenham

Lockwood Reservoir

Former site of AEC Factory

Vestry House Museum

Markfield Beam Engine and Museum

Walthamstow Reservoirs

Walthamstow

A1006

Low Hall Pump House

New River Head

Stoke Newington Pumping Station

Walthamstow Marshes

Frederick Bremer's House and Workshop

Lea Bridge Speedway Stadium

A12

A105

A104

A107

A10

R. Lee Navigation

Temple Mills Eurostar Depot

Leyton

Stoke Newington

Stratford International Station

A104

Hackney

R. Lea

Former Stratford works of the Great Eastern Railway

West Ham Park

Stratford

Grand Union Canal

Hertford Union Canal

Olympic Park

Regent's Canal

A501

Bethnal Green

Abbey Mills Pumping Station

A11

A12

Three Mills Island

Bromley – by-Bow

R. Lea

A1011

A13

Whitechapel

A13

A1203

A1011

Bow Creek Ecology Park

River Thames

West India Docks

Leamouth

East India Docks

Former Site of Thames Ironworks & Shipbuilding Co.,

0   .3 km
           .9 miles

Scale 1:20,000

© Middlesex University Press 2009